Kombucha
Rediscovered

**The Medicinal Benefits of an
Ancient Healing Tea**
Revised Edition

Klaus Kaufmann, DSc

Books Alive
Summertown, TN

D1025335

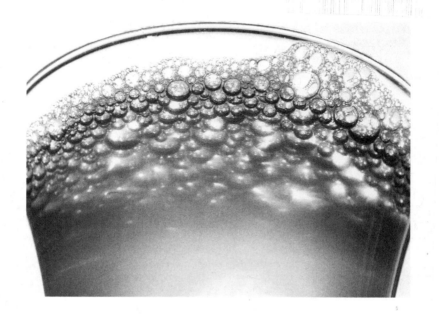

Cover and interior design: Deirdre Nemmers
Cover photography: Andrew Schmidt and Liz Murray

Books Alive, an imprint of Book Publishing Company
PO Box 99
Summertown, TN 38483
888-260-8458
bookpubco.com

ISBN 13: 978-0-920470-84-8

19 18 17 16 15 14 13   1 2 3 4 5 6 7 8 9

Printed in The United States of America
Library of Congress Cataloging-in-Publication Data

Kaufmann, Klaus N., 1942-
  Kombucha rediscovered! : the medicinal benefits of an ancient healing tea / Klaus Kaufmann. -- Revised edition.
    pages cm
Includes bibliographical references and index.
  ISBN 978-0-920470-84-8 (pbk.) -- ISBN 978-0-920470-76-3 (e-book)
  1. Kombucha tea. 2. Tea fungus--Therapeutic use. I. Title.
  RM666.T25K38 2013
  615.3'21--dc23

2012038851

Book Publishing Company is a member of Green Press Initiative. We chose to print this title on paper with 100% postconsumer recycled content, processed without chlorine, which saved the following natural resources:

- 17 trees
- 541 pounds of solid waste
- 8,077 gallons of water
- 1,489 pounds of greenhouse gases
- 7 million BTU of energy

For more information on Green Press Initiative, visit www.greenpressinitiative.org. Environmental impact estimates were made using the Environmental Defense Fund Paper Calculator. For more information visit www.papercalculator.org.

To my devoted mother, who brewed
the tastiest tea in the world.

I suppose I ought to eat or drink something or other; but the great question is, what? Alice looked all round her at the flowers and the blades of grass, but she did not see anything that looked like the right thing to eat or drink under the circumstances. There was a large mushroom growing near her, about the same height as herself; and when she had looked under it, and on both sides of it, and behind it, it occurred to her that she might as well look and see what was on the top of it.

—Lewis Carroll, *Alice's Adventures in Wonderland*

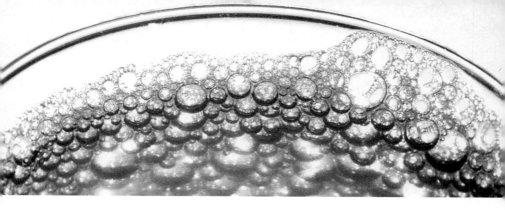

Contents

The role of the infinitely small in nature is infinitely great.

—Louis Pasteur

Foreword

Hardly a day goes by at the Wild Rose College of Natural Healing or clinic that someone doesn't phone to ask a question about kombucha tea, which callers also may refer to as "that mushroom tea" or maybe "that pancake mushroom tea." Given the current level of interest, the timing couldn't be more appropriate for an informative book about this healing tea.

Is the tea just a fad? Kombucha tea's popularity has come and gone over the centuries. Knowledge of it goes back at least two thousand years, a substantial span of time, I think, that clearly indicates that kombucha tea is here to stay. How, then, should we describe it? Is it food from the gods? Is it a panacea? Can it cure conditions as diverse as arthritis, baldness, and cancer? I hope you'll find answers to such questions, and many more, in this book.

While commercial brands of kombucha tea can be purchased in some natural food stores, the tea is most often brewed at home. With each fresh batch, a new kombucha culture or "baby" is formed, making it possible for home brewers to pass along new cultures to family members and friends. Because brewing kombucha tea involves microorganisms, careful handling of the kombucha culture is a must, as is using proven methods, like those described in this book, when making the tea at home. These are probably the most important considerations related to the tea.

Is kombucha tea safe for everyone? Many practitioners have suggested that people who have an impaired or weakened immune system should avoid the tea. Others recommend that people who have yeast infections shouldn't use the tea. In addition, some have cautioned people with diabetes against using the tea because of its potential sugar content. However, since all kombucha teas don't contain the same strains of bacteria and yeast, and because brewing time largely determines the sugar content in the final product, these concerns may apply to some teas but not to others.

I believe we'll be hearing many more reports of healing agents coming from such microorganisms as bacteria, yeast, and fungi. Although I don't believe that any medicinal substance can in itself cure an ailment, I heartily acknowledge that some substances can help us on the way to a better quality of life. This includes the medicinal use of microorganisms, which isn't a new approach. Many mainstream antibiotics, for example, were derived from microorganisms. In addition, some people introduce friendly bacteria, such as acidophilus, into their diets in the form of yogurt or supplements, because having a proper ecological balance of microorganisms in the gut can be so important in determining one's overall state of health.

As time goes on, the mystery about kombucha tea will be solved; science will reveal explanations for the tea's functional effects on human physiology. In the meantime, if you want to become a kombucha tea drinker or brewmaster, or are simply curious about what kombucha tea is, this book is a good place to start.

—Terry Willard, PhD
Wild Rose College of Natural Healing
and Wild Rose Wholistic Clinic

Publisher's Note to the First Edition

The modern age dawned and with it came the nightmare of modern food preparation. Refrigeration, pasteurization, canning, processing, and freezing may be convenient in our fast-paced society, but these methods have made our food base devoid of nutrition. All of these commonplace practices rob food of its vitamins, minerals, enzymes, and essential fatty acids. As a result, we have seen a dramatic increase in the frequency of such frightening diseases as cancer, and people are plagued with chronic diseases of the bowels, stomach, and liver. Poor nutrition—and thus poor health—has led people to search for alternative methods of food preparation. Often, these seekers simply rediscover ancient practices.

Lately, there has been renewed awareness of the benefits of lactic acid-fermented foods. Lactic acid fermentation is the oldest-known method for preserving food. To keep fruits and vegetables for the winter, our ancestors fermented them and stored them underground in storage cellars, which, unlike our modern basements, were not sealed from moisture and air. Many of the other staples in our ancestors' diets were preserved and stored in this manner. Whole, raw, and unrefined foods were stored with such fermented foods as sourdough bread, kefir, cured meats, and natural cheeses. These foods provided the nutritional foundation for an active life. Today, however, according to postindustrial perspectives about nutrition, these forms of food preparation and storage are considered primitive and tedious. Yet, such common and ancient practices can't be dismissed so easily. Luckily for us, fermented foods are coming back into fashion.

Why are fermented foods so critical for good health? The answer to this question is clear. The fermentation process has been proven to produce a variety of health-supporting substances, from acetylcholine, which benefits the body's nervous system, to choline, which normalizes blood pressure and prevents hypertension. In addition, fermented foods are rich in vitamins B and C and are full of enzymes. Unlike other methods of food preservation, lactic acid fermentation maintains the life and the nutritional value of the microorganism that's involved in the fermentation. Lactic acids, the direct products of the fermentation process, are found in such foods as yogurt and sauerkraut, and they benefit the human body in more ways than was previously imagined. "Good" lactic acid—also called L(+) lactic acid—successfully battles digestive problems by aiding the expulsion and elimination of unfriendly bacteria and cleansing the bowels. Detoxification is a key principle of optimal health, as the elimination of unnecessary substances provides the body with boundless energy and life.

The lost art of fermentation was bound to be rediscovered. Most discoveries start with a mystery in which only hints and clues are revealed. Kombucha tea, a fermented beverage, is one of these clues. Used for centuries, the tea is worthy of our attention. When kombucha tea is added to a balanced diet, the mystery of obtaining ideal health by consuming properly prepared foods and drinks is well on the way to being solved.

—Siegfried Gursche

Acknowledgments

This book is the product of two passions that have been with me throughout my life. First, I have had a love of writing since I was published and won a writer's prize when I was only ten years old. Second, I have searched for the secret to perfect health since I was misdiagnosed by orthodox medicine at the age of fourteen.

My lifelong interest in health led me to research and write the first edition of this book in the 1990s. At that time, some truly remarkable people provided me with knowledge about the kombucha culture and kombucha tea, and I want to offer my very special thanks to my 1990s kombucha gurus: Waltraut Schaffer, Wal Kneifel, Murray Mitchell, Alex Lauder, Sandra Poulton, and Peter Theiss. For this second edition, I want to acknowledge the people who have provided new and exciting insights, including Suzanne Stoeckle, Sergi Rollan, and Chantale Houle, all of Kefiplant. And last, but not least, I give my thanks to Matthew Breech of TallGrass, a distributor of kombucha products based in Vancouver, British Columbia, that's quickly conquering the Canadian health food market, for allowing me to sample all of his medicinal kombucha products.

All of these individuals contributed meaningfully either toward the "brewing" of the first edition or the "rebrewing" of the second edition of this book. Furthermore, the first edition was made possible by kombucha lover and former publisher Siegfried Gursche, while this updated version exists thanks to my new publishers, Cynthia and Bob Holzapfel, and their staff at Book Publishing Company. As always, my wife, Gabriele, who is constantly interested in what I'm up to, diligently supported my efforts, and our beautiful cat, Samedi, curled up at my feet and kept me company for hours on end.

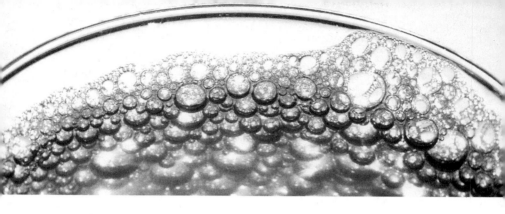

Introduction

Kombucha tea has come a long way since I initially researched the topic and published the first edition of this book. Today, there's a kombucha renaissance as commercial versions of not only the tea but also a number of spin-off products become increasingly available in North America and many other parts of the world. Another indication of kombucha tea's renewed popularity is the continued enthusiasm for brewing it at home. This ancient remedy, which emerged in Asia centuries ago, has had a steady presence in Russia and periodically reappeared during resurgences elsewhere in Europe over the past hundred years or so.

As is often the case, newer state-of-the-art research can be useful in supplementing older findings. The updated edition of this book includes the most current information I could find, which we'll explore alongside the fruits of my original research. Because kombucha tea is very ancient—rather than very new—my earlier findings largely remain relevant. By combining them with the most up-to-date information about kombucha tea, I hope to resolve any misunderstandings or misinformation that readers may have about the tea.

The early chapters of this book (see chapters 1 through 3) introduce both the kombucha culture and kombucha tea, providing details about their history as well as existing theories and published research. There's still some mystery surrounding kombucha tea, and questions remain about its effective ingredients and exactly how the tea works as a healing agent. I expect answers to these questions will be found over time. For now, we have a wealth of anecdotal evidence and a rich history on which to base our faith in kombucha tea. In chapter 4, I share information about how the tea seems to be useful for specific ailments.

A seemingly ever-increasing number of commercially brewed kombucha teas is now on the market, and many are quite different from home-brewed kombucha teas. While I include a new section in this book about the professional brews (see chapter 6), which can be quite tasty, this book is dedicated primarily to making kombucha tea at home (see chapter 5). For me, brewing the tea myself is a labor of love and a rewarding hobby.

I learned about kombucha tea when I was exploring health-related topics for my other books. After encountering many ailing and overweight people during research trips throughout the United States and Canada, I decided to write a book on juice fasting for cleansing, slimming, and health restoration. The final product was titled *The Joy of Juice Fasting*, and it was while I was writing about this topic that I first heard about kombucha tea. Fasting and cleansing are vital contributors to health and well-being, and consuming ample amounts of healthful beverages is imperative to overall health. When I discovered kombucha tea, I got a good feeling about the tea's innate restorative value for fasting, detoxifying, and last, but not least, pure drinking enjoyment.

Then, while I was studying silica for two other books that I wrote, *Silica: The Forgotten Nutrient* and *Silica: The Amazing Gel,* I observed that though we often scorn simple remedies, inspired healers throughout history, including the ancient Chinese and Greeks, used them consistently and successfully. While we might tend to think of these medicine men and women of old as having mystical powers, the reality is that they had a deep knowledge of the simple healing arts. Modern science is only now rediscovering some of these secrets. In the West in particular, science has "forgotten" and has had to "discover" and reintroduce us to many ancient healing herbs and substances. Prompted by these thoughts, I recalled the ancient healing tea.

I decided to study kombucha tea in earnest in 1990 with plans to write a self-help guide about it. When I sent out feelers on the topic, a German friend told me she had seen what she called "a wondrous mushroom" on her mother's kitchen shelf in her apartment in downtown Munich. In fact, over time, the kombucha culture has frequently been referred to as a "mushroom," so this comment by my friend isn't surprising to me now. My friend told me that,

We are talking about a "Panacea" Manchurian Mushroom that takes seven days to reproduce itself. It looks like a grayish colored hot cake. It is very fast growing and turns the tea into radical proteins, enzymes and vitamins that work to clean and detoxify your blood very quickly. Properly cultivated it is good for:

1. Eliminates wrinkles and helps removal of brown spots on hands. It's a skin humectant.
2. Prevents certain types of cancer in Manchuria, where this mushroom is from, not one case of cancer has been detected. Each day the people drink this tea as a religious atonement.
3. During menopause, reduces hot-flash discomforts. Just after drinking the tea you may feel a warm sensation, due to the fact that the teas components join the blood stream causing a draining action of toxic chemical elements and fluids, the reason for which you will notice increased mobility in your extremities and flexibility around your waist.
4. Helps with constipation.
5. Helps muscular aches and pains in the shoulders and neck.
6. Helps bronchitis, asthma, coughs in 2 days. Helps children with phlegm.
7. Helps with allergies, also with aching nerves.
8. It is prescribed in kidney problems.
9. It's proven useful in cataracts and other formations on the cornea.
10. It cleanses the gall bladder, helps colitis and nervous stomachs.
11. It helps heal diseases. It will lower cholesterol & softens veins & arteries.
12. It will stop infectious diarrhea.
13. Helps burning of fat, therefore it also helps one to lose weight.
14. Helps with insomnia.
15. Helps the liver work more efficiently.
16. Helps to level off glucose, and sudden drops of blood sugar in diabetes. Taken daily, it eliminates urea in 100 days.
17. It has surprising effects on the scalp, it helps avoid balding, thickens hair, helps to eliminate gray hair.
18. Helps digestion.
The Manchurian Mushroom has all of these miraculous properties. It was brought into Mexico from Shogegachum, Manchuria, on the Siberian border.

HOW TO PREPARE YOUR TEA AND PROPAGATE THE MUSHROOM

You must use a glass or enameled pot or container (3 1/2 quart glass pot by Visions is ideal) there can be no metal rim. When you handle the mushroom, take off all of your rings and any other metal that could come into near proximity to the mushroom. If you use a spoon be sure it is wooden plastic or ceramic.

Heat 3 quarts of water, when it starts to boil add I cup of

SPRING WATER or Distilled # 1-CUP 5 TEA BAG LET STEEP

3   Introduction

oddly enough, she had failed to ask her mother about "that thing" floating in a brownish liquid, and her mother never offered her any explanations about it either. Years later, after my friend had moved to Canada, an acquaintance gave her a similar "mushroom," urging it on her as a great cure-all. The acquaintance referred to it as the "Manchurian," and with it she gave my friend a hand-me-down leaflet on how to cultivate this "Manchurian." As I later discovered, "Manchurian mushroom" is another popular name for the kombucha culture.

When my friend showed me the old leaflet, I found its fragmentary instructions so powerful that I decided to reproduce the leaflet in this book (see page 3). As you can see, someone added the handwritten notes at the bottom and the whole thing was typed on an old typewriter, complete with spelling errors and obvious omissions. To retain the charm and authenticity, the reproduction contains all the original errors.

But was this the kombucha I was looking for? My friend told me she kept it in her refrigerator and had stopped drinking the tea. She also had never heard the word "kombucha," and she couldn't confirm whether her "mushroom" could be the kombucha culture. Remarkably, she did tell me that a biochemist at the University of British Columbia in Vancouver had analyzed this "Manchurian" for the acquaintance who gave it to her. The biochemist had confirmed that the culture was biologically active and contained healthful components, just as the leaflet asserted. I contacted the university in hopes of speaking with the biochemist myself, but I couldn't find him at the time and suspected he had transferred to another university. Nonetheless, I appeared to be on the right track regarding my kombucha research.

Before long I knew I had been given a true kombucha culture, and as I traced the history of kombucha tea, I discovered that the "Manchurian" wasn't new at all and was actually quite ancient. Yet, it's clear that kombucha tea was at times forgotten. Indeed, catastrophic events—such as two world wars—can force people to focus on momentary survival, and at such times, ancient health secrets can be forgotten.

In today's scientifically advanced world, better hygiene, nutrition, and health care have resulted in ever-increasing longevity. Suddenly, there's a dire necessity to stay well and productive into our seventies, eighties, nineties, and even our hundreds, and Western governments can no longer afford to provide adequate health care or retirement benefits for aging populations. There's little wonder that people are searching for ways to take control and maintain their own health while avoiding orthodox or expensive medical treatments. In such circumstances, remedies like kombucha tea seem to come back just in the nick of time. Indeed, the tea can be considered a tonic, taken routinely to bolster good health, rather than as a treatment for any particular disease.

And yet, some practitioners have sworn by the tea in treating certain ailments, including cancer, and this isn't surprising. While researching alternative treatments for cancer, I noticed that health-bestowing foods containing fermented sauerkraut and fermented juices are extremely important. They're essential, I realized, not only for those who suffer from cancer, but also for all who are delivering health care (in the best sense of that word) to ourselves, our families, our friends, and our neighbors—in short, to all of us. A fermented beverage, kombucha tea is as valuable as these other fermented foods and drinks.

As I stated earlier, this book combines old and new research to best answer any questions that you may have about kombucha tea. I invite you to think of this book as a revival of ancient lore. Healers created and used kombucha tea centuries ago. They knew more about the friendly and beneficial coexistence (symbiosis) of microscopic life forms and their influence on human health than even modern researchers.

I began this introduction with a favorite quote from *Alice's Adventures in Wonderland*. Just as poor Alice becomes lost, I believe humanity has lost many of its health-wise ways over the eons. Also much like Alice, we need someone to remind us from time to time of the good things. Anyone who is familiar with this classic tale knows of the mushroom that Alice ate in response to the caterpillar's advice. I suppose that, in a way, this book is like the direction-giving caterpillar, and I hope you'll find it a valuable guide. (Although I advise against smoking the pipe, especially since tobacco smoke can damage the kombucha culture.)

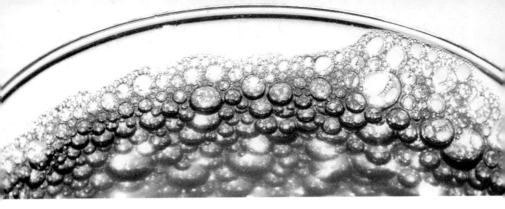

Chapter One

Introducing Kombucha

I received my first kombucha culture from Sandra Poulton in 1995, the year the first edition of this book came out. I lived in Vancouver, British Columbia, and Poulton lived in Lion's Head, Ontario. She secured my kombucha "baby" in a plastic bag, floated it in some kombucha tea, and sent it to me via courier. Two days later, I saw my first kombucha culture.

I'll never forget the great taste experience I had the day my initial batch of kombucha tea was ready. I shut my eyes and kept them tightly closed as I guzzled down the very first glass. I had tasted only the tiniest bit of the cider-like liquid that came with the kombucha culture, so I was totally unprepared to discover that my fresh kombucha tea tasted just like French bubbly.

Although I didn't know it at the time, my first taste of home-brewed kombucha tea was typical. When it has fermented for about seven days and is freshly harvested, the tea tastes like sweet champagne. After it has been stored in the refrigerator, the tea tastes similar to other fermented drinks, such as wine or beer, or nonalcoholic beverages. For example, Poulton, who got her first kombucha culture from a friend, compares the taste to apple cider. Others liken the effervescent tea to cola.

While kombucha tea may remind some users of alcoholic beverages, the tea has very little alcohol (about .5 percent). It also doesn't contain the damaging amount of sugar that's typically found in commercial drinks, and although it contains a small amount of caffeine, it's minimal and comparable to what is in a cup of decaffeinated coffee. Because people generally like a tongue-tingling fizz and sweetness, beverage manufacturers deliver both (and bolster sales) by carbonating commercial drinks and adding excessive amounts of sugar. Most people love sugar and believe they can't live without it, but those who wish to limit their sugar intake have a friend in kombucha tea. The tea is simultaneously refreshing, energizing, and extraordinarily healthful, with no added sweetener necessary. People enjoy drinking it because it's naturally fizzy and tastes great. The tea also soothes the stomach within minutes of drinking it.

If you, like me, enjoy a healthful, thirst-quenching drink, come on board. If you've been searching for a magic potion that's rejuvenating and tastes wonderful, you can end your search today. Kombucha tea will keep you healthy and satisfied, without causing cravings or unwanted side effects.

FAQ

Q: What is the alcohol content of kombucha tea?

A: The amount of alcohol in home-brewed kombucha tea is very low, usually just above .5 percent for teas that have fermented for ten days. The percentage is even lower for teas that have fermented for less time. Teas that are left to ferment longer than ten days have 1 to 2 percent alcohol content. You might think you can increase the alcohol content of the tea by adding more sugar, but don't try it. Adding more sugar will make the tea too acidic since the alcohol in the tea is converted into vinegar.

The Living Food You Can Drink

Kombucha tea is a probiotic, which means that it contains living microorganisms that confer a health benefit on their host. (*Probiotic* means "for life.") Kombucha tea, like other living foods, also contains acids, enzymes, and vitamins that have been associated with myriad health benefits. The tea is particularly known to aid digestion, boost energy, and strengthen the immune system. (See chapter 3 for more information about the powerful contents of kombucha tea and chapter 4 to explore some of the reported health benefits.)

Kombucha tea is the result of a fermentation process. When the tea is left to ferment for seven days or longer, microbes in the kombucha culture release enzymes that create complex changes. Microbial fermentation is a natural process that has been around for centuries. Ancient people made yogurt and butter using this process, for example. Alcohol is also derived from a fermentation process in which yeast ferments grape juice into wine and barley into beer and whiskey.

So what is kombucha tea composed of? As described in chapter 5, only a few ingredients are needed: the kombucha culture, tea, purified water, and white sugar. By the time the tea is ready to drink, however, very little sugar remains. That's because the kombucha culture is a colony of helpful bacteria and yeast that grows in a medium of cellulose, and the bacteria and yeast consume and convert the sugar during fermentation. (The kombucha culture is similar to a yogurt culture or kefir culture that ferments in milk.)

The kombucha culture looks like a pancake or mushroom. In fact, mainly for the sake of convenience, the kombucha culture is often called a mushroom. It does, after all, "mushroom," or grow quickly, so it's aptly named, although a kombucha isn't really a mushroom in the proper biological sense. Those who wish to avoid the term "mushroom" refer to the culture as a "SCOBY," which is an acronym for "symbiotic colony of bacteria and yeast."

The symbiotic partners profit from each other. The yeast delivers the food that the bacteria need to grow, and the bacteria protect the yeast. On their own, neither could continue to exist for long. Here's an overview of the process: During fermentation, the yeast cells in the kombucha culture busily feed on the nutrients provided by the sugar and the tea. As a result of this metabolism, the yeast cells change the sugar to ethyl alcohol (ethanol) and carbon dioxide. The bacteria begin to flourish and convert the alcohol into acetic acid, or vinegar, and other organic acids. The kombucha tea is increasingly soured, and the alcohol acts as a poison for disease-causing germs, which can't survive in the tea.

Meanwhile, the bacteria change the sugar into cellulose. This process allows the kombucha culture floating on top of the tea to grow, and a second kombucha culture takes shape. So every time you ferment a batch of kombucha tea, the original kombucha culture, sometimes referred to as the kombucha "mother," gives birth to a baby that you can use yourself or pass along to a friend or family member who may be interested in the benefits of kombucha tea.

Kombucha tea has traditionally been brewed at home by people who have enjoyed its taste along with its ability to quench thirst and bolster health. Today, kombucha tea and related products are also widely available from commercial manufacturers. If you're not yet ready to make kombucha tea yourself, go to the local natural food store and sample some of the products you find there. (See chapter 6 for my impressions about some of the commercial brews that are currently available.)

Praised by Users

I first heard about kombucha tea from my friend Waltraut Schaffer, who brought it from Germany and made it to treat her digestive troubles. According to Schaffer, her digestion promptly improved after she began drinking kombucha tea. Initially, she was a little concerned about the sugar in the tea, but as we now know, after fermentation, very little sugar remains in the tea.

Sandra Poulton, who gave me my first kombucha baby, drinks kombucha tea mainly to keep up her program of preventive health care. She says, "I drink kombucha for its health-bestowing properties. I have a general concern to stay healthy." She adds, "I don't have any major problems right now, and I don't want any!"

Like Poulton, I was initially interested in kombucha tea for maintaining health. Fermenting kombucha tea for longer times dramatically improves this potential but also intensifies the flavor. As Poulton cautions, "The taste might be a bit overwhelming for newcomers to kombucha because it can be quite sharp. Yet, if you can drink apple cider vinegar, you can drink kombucha tea."

In the book *Kombucha Phenomenon,* writers Betsy Pryor and Sanford Holst flood readers with impressive testimonials from kombucha drinkers from all over the United States. I heard Pryor speak in Las Vegas, Nevada, during a National Nutritional Foods Association convention. Pryor related how, at age forty-nine, she lost fourteen pounds after drinking kombucha tea for two months. Though she didn't work out much, her muscles became firmer. Then after one year of drinking kombucha tea, she noticed her gray hairs were regaining color. When she had been drinking kombucha tea for two years, her hair thickened and was longer than ever. In addition, she reported sleeping less but being more focused. She also noticed that she was developing a photographic memory. All sound like good reasons for kombucha tea to become the drink of choice for some Hollywood actors, whom Pryor says use it instead of artificial stimulants to sustain them through grueling sixteen-hour workdays.

Attendees of Pryor's presentation offered their own testimonials, discussing what they gained from drinking kombucha tea. Here are some typical comments:

"My complexion cleared up."

"I've lost weight. I just want to eat less."

"I have better digestion, and I really feel it has helped my liver."

"I sleep less but more soundly. And I have more energy throughout the day."

"It helps me with my menopause. It just balances me through the hot flashes—I'm just sliding through it."

One attendee discussed how her son, who works in construction, uses the tea to quench his thirst on hot days: "My son says he can drink a full glass of kombucha tea on the job and have his thirst quenched, or he can drink a gallon of water and feel terrible afterward." Another mother noted that her twenty-six-year-old son is using the tea to combat baldness: "I've had my son on it now about four months. He told me, 'Mom, I'm getting hair! My hair is coming back!'"

I came across one additional testimonial that I'd like to include here. In the Dutch magazine *Op Zoek,* a fifteen-year-old boy from the Netherlands recalled his experience with kombucha tea: "The misery began when I was ten years old, and it lasted four years. At first the itching began in my arms, and I scratched them till they bled, especially in bed at night. After six weeks I went to the doctor. I was given a course of penicillin and ointment, because one arm was inflamed from the scratching. This lasted for about a year and a half. I kept getting more ointment, one lot after the other, and it was the same with the penicillin. Finally, I had to go to a hospital specialist. The doctor talked about some intestinal bacteria that were the cause of the trouble. Then I was given more medicine, which made me feel numb, but the itching remained . . . but now my mother's been making kombucha tea for the past six months. I began drinking it right away, and after only one week the itching was gone. I feel as if

I've been born again. Even the scars are hardly visible anymore. I'd like to tell everybody to stop taking medicine and drink kombucha."

Prescribed by Professionals

In addition to hearing from the users of kombucha tea, I spoke with professionals who recommend the tea to their clients. Wanting to learn more about its practical applications, I discussed kombucha tea with Bonnie Mori, who is an acupuncturist, certified herbalist, and student of Chinese medicine in Niagara-on-the-Lake, Ontario. She says, "Besides drinking it regularly myself, I prescribe kombucha tea to my clients for many conditions and, invariably, they meet with success. I have also recommended it to my entire family and friends for digestive ailments, including constipation, belching, and gas, and for lack of energy. I have even given the tea to my cats and dogs, and I find that they're less prone to infections."

Mori describes some of the positive effects of kombucha tea: "I have given it to a client with diabetes to treat her diarrhea. It worked and she even obtained some desired weight loss. I also know of at least one person who, besides drinking it regularly, used kombucha tea as an astringent. This person successfully combated acne and claims to have less oily hair." Mori also recounts a story about another case she treated with kombucha tea: "This fellow burped all night and couldn't sleep a wink. The burping stopped, and he sleeps like a baby."

Mori says that it's typical for clients who use kombucha tea to comment that they look younger than ever. She adds that those who use the tea also confirm having much more energy. As Mori puts it, "Some people get instantaneously more energy after drinking kombucha tea, and that energy is sustained for the rest of the day. For instance, I gave the tea to a top corporate manager who is living in my area. He likes to play hockey as a counterbalance to his sedentary occupation, but his game had slackened off. Now he has enough energy for two games."

Mori thinks kombucha tea acts as a catalyst in the body, causing numerous beneficial changes over time. She says the energizing effect that people notice almost immediately is due to the amino acids and the vitamins in the tea, which are instantaneously absorbed.

Many of Mori's clients are a bit sheepish about adopting a kombucha baby and starting to brew the tea at home. Because they're afraid of other people's reactions or opinions, they say, "I can't believe that I'm taking this home!" However, once they start drinking the tea and experiencing the health benefits, they're hooked. Over time, they even begin to pass along the tea to their family, friends, and neighbors.

Kombucha tea has also found acceptance in the well-respected discipline of homeopathy. Alex Lauder of Guelph, Ontario, is a homeopathic practitioner who uses kombucha tea in his practice. Lauder recommends kombucha tea to his patients mainly as an adjunct to a multidisciplinary homeopathic program for cancer treatment. Lauder says, "As part of the program and whenever patients need antioxidants, I suggest kombucha tea. I know of cases in which remission occurred that could only be ascribed to the kombucha. We have seen lumps disappear from under the skin of kombucha users."

Lauder emphasizes that he provides the kombucha tea free of charge to his patients and that there's no profit motive involved in his kombucha treatment. Kombucha tea can be made at low cost. With the possible exception of commercial manufacturers (see chapter 6), nobody makes a fortune off kombucha tea. To me, this fact underscores its genuine usefulness as a remedy.

Lauder says his wife drinks kombucha tea and also uses it regularly on her face. He confirms that her skin looks younger than ever and that her facial lines have disappeared.

Known in Military and Athletic Circles

According to writer and researcher Harald Tietze, members of the Russian military are regularly given kombucha tea to drink. He also reports that kombucha tea usage has been studied by the German military. Under the direction of Simon Gerrit, researchers at the military-operated sports school concluded, "Pure biological kombucha fermented tea has a strengthening effect and improves the performance of the athletes."

Additional research results from Germany confirm that drinking kombucha tea can be of benefit to athletes. At the Olympic training ground in Warendorf, researchers tested twelve trained athletes who drank about seven fluid ounces (about 200 milliliters) of kombucha tea per day. Blood tests confirmed that the athletes achieved better training times after consuming the kombucha tea. The athletes also felt more energetic and recovered more quickly when they drank kombucha tea. The researchers concluded that drinking kombucha tea led to positive changes in the energy metabolism of the cells, which could explain the increased physical abilities and enhanced well-being the athletes experienced. The use of kombucha tea among athletes has been observed in other parts of Europe as well. In Russia, for example, trainers give kombucha tea to high-performance athletes to increase their energy output.

There have even been reports in European health magazines about kombucha tea being given to camels that are used for racing in Arab countries. The total composition of the camel "dope," however, was kept a proprietary secret.

A Healthful Thirst Quencher for Children

Rosina Fasching, perhaps the most famous kombucha researcher and writer, and a number of other researchers recommend kombucha tea as a drink for children. Fasching's only caution is that kombucha tea usually contains a bit of caffeine, which could stimulate children. To make kombucha tea more palatable for youngsters, it can easily be diluted with their favorite fruit juice or water.

Kombucha Tea and the Future

When I moved into a new home some years back, I discovered a stone sculpture in the otherwise empty house. The sculpture depicted the number one hundred. I was delighted because the year of the move was also the year of my fiftieth birthday. I interpreted the sculpture as a positive sign that I'll reach the age of one hundred, when I plan to be traveling, gardening, and writing my memoirs. I'm hopeful that drinking kombucha tea will help me attain these goals. After all, drinking the tea is already famously associated with longevity in the Kargasok region of Russia (where it's called "Kargasok tea"). The people there drink the tea throughout their lives.

While drinking kombucha tea has long been a tradition in the Kargasok region, I wouldn't be surprised if it became a much more common practice around the globe. As the population increases and the world's resources are stretched, rediscovering ancient methods of food preparation will no doubt become increasingly more important. Fermented beverages, such as kombucha tea and kefir, are now accepted in the mainstream as healthful drinks, and they may become much more prevalent in the future.

Although we still await scientific explanations about the healing properties of kombucha tea, there are two important points to remember. First, testimonials clearly indicate that kombucha tea aids digestion and detoxification, increasing overall energy. Second, kombucha tea provides an inexpensive and delicious alternative to alcoholic and carbonated beverages, which are loaded with sugar and preservatives. With kombucha tea in hand, we'll be able to face the future with enthusiasm and cheer.

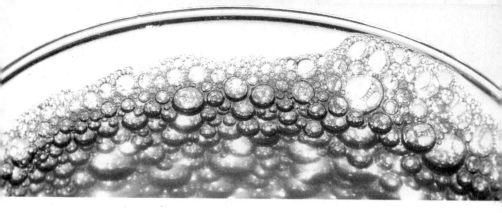

Chapter Two
Kombucha's Illustrious Past and Promise

Although we don't know exactly how or where the kombucha culture originated, all signs point to the East. According to author Günther Frank, the first recorded use of kombucha tea was in ancient China. In the year 221 BC, during the Tsin Dynasty, kombucha was hailed as "the tea of immortality." Today, the tea remains a favorite folk remedy in China. Research by Sergi Rollan, a medical doctor, research biologist, and nutritionist associated with Kefiplant, also suggests that kombucha came from the Far East, probably China. Another possible point of origin is Caucasia, the region where Asia and Europe meet, between the Black and Caspian Seas.

Author Betsy Pryor holds that the kombucha culture may have originated in the Middle East and made its way to Europe and America via the Far East. She believes kombucha contains some lichen, a source of antibacterial usnic acid, which is a major constituent of manna according to some theories. Described in the Bible as feeding the children of Israel, manna is known as "food from heaven." Pryor suggests that kombucha was carried along the traditional spice routes that existed between the Mediterranean and the Far East. Kombucha tea would have been a popular beverage because it took months for caravans to traverse the route, and travelers would have needed fermented foods that wouldn't spoil.

Over the years, there has been debate not only about where the kombucha culture came from, but also about what it is. According to Helmut Golz, a German physician who has written a book about kombucha, the culture was once thought to be a sponge that was fished from the sea; its curative properties were ascribed to its iodine content. Others, including researchers from the Central Bacteriological Institute in Moscow, declared the kombucha culture to be a lichen. A symbiosis of algae and fungi, lichens originated some 2.5 million years ago. However, while lichens are recognized for their healing properties, they require light for photosynthesis, whereas the kombucha culture happily grows in total darkness. As we now know, Western science has established the kombucha culture to be neither a lichen nor a sponge, but rather a symbiosis of bacteria and yeast cells.

Kombucha Arrives in the West

By the turn of the twentieth century, kombucha had traveled west from Mongolia and Russia and became known in other parts of Europe. In 1913, sources described kombucha for the first time in German literature. A kombucha coming from Russia was discussed: "They employed it against all kind of ailments."

Kombucha tea has had a steady presence in Russia, where the home-brewed drink continues to thrive as a folk remedy today. The kombucha culture was also used to make a popular kvass, a sour beer-like beverage made of rye meal, malt, and other ingredients, including spices. From Russia, the kvass made its way into Poland during World War I. Records mention a Polish apothecary who prepared a laxative based on a "Russian secret recipe." By 1914, residents of Prague had heard of kombucha tea. After World War I, kombucha tea made a comeback first in Denmark and then in the German province of East Prussia. Returning German prisoners of war carried the kombucha culture to Stettin and Saxony. By 1927, some people in Westphalia and Hamburg knew kombucha tea as a home remedy.

Following World War II, kombucha tea became known primarily in Italy but also in France and Spain. Surprisingly, it had clearly been forgotten in Germany at that time. We don't know why kombucha tea has gone through periods of relative renown and obscurity; my theory is that people forgot kombucha because of the pressing business of daily survival. It's also possible that the tradition of brewing kombucha tea died out during the war years and afterward because so many staples, including sugar, were rationed. At the time, who could afford to feed precious sugar to a symbiotic culture?

By the 1960s, kombucha tea saw a renaissance in Germany through the work of Rudolf Sklenar, a medical practitioner who used the tea extensively to treat cancer patients. Sklenar also prescribed the tea for metabolic disorders, rheumatism, gout, high blood pressure, high cholesterol, and diabetes. He recorded various successes in these areas but was particularly concerned about cancer. He frowned upon orthodox cancer treatments, such as surgery and chemotherapy, and preferred biological therapies for prevention and healing. Apparently, Sklenar's method was also practiced by Veronika Carstens, a medical doctor who was married to the former West German president. In her writings from the 1980s, Carstens mentioned kombucha tea.

A Kombucha by Any Other Name

The word kombucha is said to be derived from the Japanese terms "kombu" (brown algae) and "cha" (tea). Another theory is that the name refers to a Korean physician by the name of Kombu, who allegedly treated the Japanese Emperor Inkyo with the cultured tea as long ago as 415 AD.

My own research revealed more than one hundred terms in multiple languages that refer to the kombucha culture and tea. Examples include algae fungus, Indian wine fungus, Japanese sponge, Manchurian mushroom, and many others. Kombucha must have impressed folks all over the world to have earned such fanciful names. I believe this proliferation of names in and of itself is a good indication of the tea's true worth. If it had not tasted so refreshing, if it had not worked to restore health, I suspect kombucha tea wouldn't have garnered so many appellations.

Kombucha in Practice and Research

Even though the spotlight hasn't always been on kombucha, the tea was steadily used and studied by a number of European scientists and physicians during the early decades of the twentieth century. Author Günther Frank tells us that by 1914, a researcher named Bacinskaya found the beverage effective in regulating the intestinal tract. Frank also reports that in 1917, Rudolf Kobert recalled an infallible cure for rheumatism prepared from the kombucha culture, and Wilhelm Henneberg found that Russian tea kvass combated "all kinds of illness, especially constipation."

In 1927, a researcher writing in *Biological Method of Healing* reported that the kombucha culture and its metabolic products affect the regeneration of cell walls, thereby making it an excellent remedy for "hardening of the arteries," or arteriosclerosis. According to writer Tom Valentine, in 1928, a physician named Maxim Bing found kombucha tea to be a "very effective means of combating hardening of the arteries, gout, and sluggishness of the bowels." Bing also noted favorable outcomes when using kombucha tea to treat "the kidneys and the capillary vessels of the brain." In 1929, a physician named E. Arauner stated that the kombucha culture is the "most effective natural folk remedy for fatigue, lassitude, nervous tension, incipient signs of old age, hardening of the arteries, sluggishness of the bowels, gout, rheumatism, hemorrhoids, and diabetes."

Around 1929, a research team in Prague led by physician Siegwart Hermann used cats in an experiment involving kombucha. The researchers injected the cats with a cholesterol-like compound to increase the cats' blood pressure and cholesterol levels. Their goal was to test kombucha's detoxifying powers on arteriosclerosis, which leads to heart attacks or strokes in both cats and humans. The cats' cholesterol levels were thirteen times greater than normal, yet Hermann's team found that the cats who were given kombucha could tolerate the high levels, leading them to conclude that the kombucha helped the cats cope with raised cholesterol and blood pressure levels. However, the researchers cautioned that the results didn't necessarily predict human outcomes.

In another experiment, this one using rabbits, Hermann's team tested the effects of gluconic acid (a constituent of fermented kombucha tea) and found that it dissolved the rabbits' bladder stones. In Russia, other tests done with rabbits showed that kombucha tincture could be used to successfully treat infections of the cornea. Similar treatment of human conjunctivitis was equally successful.

Research in Russia demonstrated the effectiveness of using kombucha tea in treating babies and toddlers. In Moscow, researchers successfully healed stomatitis (inflammatory disease of the mouth) in toddlers, who were given kombucha tea to drink and whose mouths were rinsed with the tea. Within five days, the subjects were healed. In Omsk, babies who were suffering from dysentery were treated exclusively with kombucha tea. After one week of therapy, the subjects' symptoms receded and the dysentery-causing bacteria could no longer be found in their stool.

Also in Omsk, patients with purulent tonsillitis (which is characterized by pus and discharge) were treated with kombucha tea. The treatment entailed gargling up to ten times a day with kombucha tea and rinsing the mouth for up to fifteen minutes. The tonsillitis cleared up, and in some cases, chronic paranasal sinusitis and bowel ailments also improved. At the same clinic, patients with high blood pressure and arteriosclerosis were treated with kombucha tea. After three weeks, the clinic recorded an improvement in symptoms and a noticeable lowering of cholesterol levels.

In Moscow, tests done with mice showed that kombucha successfully activated the immune system. Mice who were given kombucha extract twenty-four hours before being exposed to a bacterial infection had an 80 percent higher survival rate than mice in the control group. Other tests showed a stimulative effect on the pituitary-adrenal cortex system.

Modern studies done by Reinhold Wiesner, a medical doctor in Schwanewede, Lower Saxony, Germany, have confirmed the antibiotic properties in kombucha tea. In a study that compared kombucha tea with an interferon preparation, Wiesner showed that the tea is comparably effective in treating certain illnesses. The test involved 250 subjects suffering from a variety of ailments, including rheumatism, kidney disease, and asthma. For the subjects with asthma, kombucha tea was considerably more effective than the interferon preparation.

Major Uses and Health Benefits

History has recorded the many therapeutic benefits of drinking kombucha tea. However, because the uses are so varied, there has been a tendency to recommend kombucha tea for all disease states. Have the tea's effects been overgeneralized? Some critics believe so, and they say it's dishonest to make medical claims about kombucha tea. In response, some writers have shied away from describing kombucha tea's beneficial effects. I, however, object to this criticism. The way I see it, few people profit from selling the tea (the home brew, in particular), so I see nothing misleading in sharing information about the tea's major uses and health benefits. I'll address some general information here; for details about specific ailments, see chapter 4.

Most likely, the greatest overall benefits from drinking kombucha tea come from its cleansing and detoxifying effects. In addition, kombucha tea, like tea in general, is rich in polyphenols, one of nature's most potent and active antioxidants, which are well affirmed to improve health status. Antioxidants provide powerful protection against free radicals, which cause oxidation, or oxidative stress, in the body. Free radicals trigger aging and chronic conditions, such as heart disease and cancer, while antioxidants are known to combat the oxidative stress associated with nearly every degenerative disease. Antioxidants are also associated with cell maintenance, DNA repair, and overall longevity.

Many kombucha experts recommend kombucha tea as a diuretic (a substance that tends to increase the elimination of urine). Therefore, people who have edemas (swelling and fluid collection), arteriosclerosis, gout, sluggish bowels, or kidney stones can benefit from drinking kombucha tea. Experts also praise kombucha tea for its ability to boost metabolism and normalize cell membranes, both of which increase overall well-being. In addition, kombucha tea is known for its ability to regulate intestinal flora, function as a natural antibiotic, and foster the acid-alkaline balance of the body. Finally, according to testimonials and expert findings, drinking kombucha tea strengthens the immune response.

A written exchange with Peter Theiss from Germany's Institute for Research of New Therapy Methods for Chronic Diseases and Immunology revealed kombucha's potential for stimulating the immune response. He writes: "Kombucha contains numerous valuable substances for the immune system and has in addition an antibiotic effect, which has been proven to act against viruses and fungi. At the same time, it enhances the defense of the body and improves defense cells, thereby improving general resistance to various infections. The phagocytes are activated and eliminate possible infectious substances within the first second after contact. Normally, a phagocyte destroys one to three particles; upon stimulation, such as by kombucha, eight to nine. Thus, the defense system is improved, and a possible illness is often prevented from breaking out altogether."

Slim and Feeling Great, Thanks to Kombucha

Being slim and feeling great often go hand in hand. Although people who are overweight may be stereotypically characterized as jolly, their weight makes them prone to blood pressure problems, diabetes, and numerous other conditions they no doubt would prefer to avoid. At the same time, they likely yearn for an improved physical appearance.

So what exactly keeps a slim person slim and an overweight person overweight? Diet and habit are contributors, certainly, but for some people, weight gain can be triggered by a malfunctioning appestat (the biological switch for controlling appetite messages between the brain and stomach). Metabolic disorders then play a large role in being overweight. By fostering metabolic healing, kombucha tea can make users feel more energized, and therefore far more likely to engage in regular physical exercise. As the saying goes, "no pain, no gain."

Those who are worried about their weight may be wondering whether kombucha tea is fattening. The caloric values of kombucha tea are difficult to establish with any accuracy. However, author Günther Frank made an attempt at calculating the calories in the tea. He found that the sugar content in the fermented tea is minimal, as is the calorie content. Here are his calculations: If about 2.5 ounces (70 grams) of white sugar is used to ferment 1 quart (roughly 1 liter) of tea, that represents about 276 calories. Of course, the fermentation process uses up a great portion of the sugar. If the remaining amount of white sugar equals about 1 ounce (30 grams), that leaves about 118 calories in 1 quart (roughly 1 liter) of tea. However, if the tea ferments longer and only .7 ounce (20 grams) of white sugar remains, that leaves about 79 calories in 1 quart (roughly 1 liter) of tea. In comparison, the same amount of cola contains *five times* the number of calories. That is that, folks.

If you want to lose weight, drinking a glass of kombucha tea ten minutes after every meal can stimulate your digestive tract. This is one method you can use to lose weight without fasting. Yet anyone can fast easily and pleasantly with the aid of kombucha tea and other fermented liquids. In my book *The Joy of Juice Fasting*, I explain the beauty and rewards of fasting. I recommend this book to users of kombucha tea who want to undertake a guided day-by-day cleansing fast using the tea.

Counting Calories for Weight Loss

In general, a daily intake of 2,500 calories is recommended for young adults and men and 2,000 calories for women. An individual's specific needs can be determined by considering other important variables, such as age, lifestyle, and physical activity. If you're curious about your daily caloric needs, why not try using an online tool? Just visit freedieting.com/tools/calorie_calculator.htm and enter your age, weight, height, gender, and exercise level to get a personalized recommendation.

Kombucha Heals the Outside Too

Now that we've discussed some of the advantages of drinking kombucha tea, let's also explore reports about kombucha tea's usefulness when applied directly to the skin. As homeopath Alex Lauder shared with me, using the tea topically can result in beautiful, wrinkle-free skin. This is a boon that kombucha tea seems to share with nutrient silica gel, a substance I have written extensively about. Nutrient silica gel, also known as *silicea*, is derived from crystals. Unlike desiccant silica, which is used for industrial purposes, nutrient silica gel is a nutrient-rich and health-supporting essential mineral, and I believe that any thorough skin-care program using kombucha tea should also incorporate nutrient silica gel.

I agree with well-known healers and herbalists, such as Rudolf Breuss, Maria Treben, and Rudolf Fritz Weiss, who maintain that the skin can absorb healing substances, including kombucha tea and nutrient silica gel. These experts have recommended taking beauty baths with kombucha tea. What could be more relaxing than enjoying a cleansing bath while simultaneously encouraging gentle healing? Simply pour a batch of fresh kombucha tea into your next bath. But why stop there? Consider using the tea on your hair too, especially if you're older. As kombucha researcher Rosina Fasching says, "With elderly people, kombucha has a rejuvenating effect, causing hair to grow in dark again." She also acknowledges the tea's ability to tighten the skin and even keep the teeth healthy.

Kombucha tea also can be used to create compresses and poultices to treat skin conditions. Wounds, ulcers, skin eruptions, injuries to muscle tissue, rheumatic pain, and fevers all respond well to external applications of kombucha tea. The pancake-like culture itself can be put into a blender and made into a cream to be used on the skin, although I recommend enlisting the help of a skilled naturopath before using this cream to dress skin conditions.

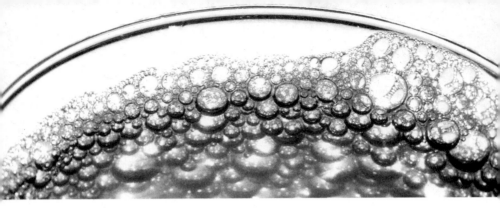

Chapter Three
A Closer Look at Kombucha

Raising a kombucha is like taking a minicourse in microbiology (the study of microscopic life forms). The kombucha culture is a conglomeration of living microorganisms, including bacteria and yeast. If this doesn't sound appetizing, stop and think for a moment about the many other types of food and drink that are made using living cultures.

Perhaps we should put the emphasis first on drinks: humankind has made beer for millennia, and yeast has always been integral in the brewing process. The same is also true for wine and most other forms of alcohol. In winemaking, the grape juice (called "must") is fermented by yeast, such as *Saccharomyces cerevisiae*. Cider and Japanese sake are other examples of culture ferments. As we know, the fermenting results in pleasant drinks that are popular the world over. The fermented kombucha beverage is equally tasty. It also is inexpensive (costing no more than a regular cup of tea), easy to make, and a worthwhile remedy if made and used correctly.

Similarly, since time immemorial, people have made yogurt, cheeses, kefir (check out my book *Kefir Rediscovered!*), and sourdough breads with yeast and bacterial cultures. Many people eat and enjoy yogurt without stopping to think that they're consuming live bacteria. Yet, these living foods are essential to our well-being. Without the aid of friendly microbes, humans and all other life forms couldn't survive for long.

This may seem counterintuitive, given that we're dreadfully afraid of bacterial infection, and rightly so. However, many friendly bacteria, such as lactobacilli and bifidobacteria, provide long-lasting health benefits when added to the diet. The microorganisms in kombucha tea also fall into this category. They're friendly and aren't out to harm us.

Beneficial Symbiosis

In chapter 1, we looked briefly at the beneficial symbiosis between the yeast and bacteria in the kombucha culture, but there's more to the story that's worth exploring. By definition, a symbiosis is a permanent or long-term association of organisms living together for mutual benefit. Symbiosis is a widespread natural phenomenon. One example is the lichen, which is a symbiosis of algae and fungi. Both organisms gain from the arrangement, with the algae providing food and vitamins through photosynthesis and the fungi providing protection from the environment.

Another compelling example of a beneficial symbiosis involves termites, insects that eat wood. They eat the wood, but they can't digest it. For this, they rely on tiny protozoans that live in their intestines. If a termite is somehow deprived of these protozoans, it starves to death, no matter how much wood it may consume.

Like these other symbiotic partners, the yeast and bacteria in the kombucha culture live together for their own mutual benefit. The yeast cells eat the sugar in the tea and change it to ethyl alcohol (ethanol) and carbon dioxide. The bacteria ferment the alcohol manufactured by the yeast cells into acetic acid and other organic acids. This means the kombucha tea is increasingly soured. During fermentation, disease-causing germs can't survive in the highly acidic kombucha tea; however, the yeast is able to survive these conditions. In other words, the bacteria protect the yeast, and in turn the yeast deliver the food on which the bacteria can grow. The partners profit from each other. On their own, neither could continue to exist for long, nor produce the health benefits for the people who drink kombucha tea.

Bacteria and Yeast in Kombucha Cultures

The partners in a kombucha symbiosis vary by region. This means that different kombucha cultures, depending on where they originated, contain different types of bacteria and yeast. This leads to interesting distinctions in the taste of the tea, and it can be fun to experiment with kombucha cultures from a number of regions. I have two strains going now, for example, and they taste slightly different.

The scientific literature describes the following main components of the symbiosis: the bacterium *Acetobacter xylinum* and the yeast *Schizosaccharomyces pombe*. In addition, researcher and author Günther Frank has identified the following bacteria and yeast strains in kombucha samples: *Bacterium xylinoides*, *Bacterium gluconicum*, *Saccharomyces ludwigii*, *Saccharomyces apiculatus*, and *Pichia fermentans*. According to researcher Helmut Golz, other bacteria and yeast strains that can be found in a kombucha culture include *Gluconobacter bluconicum*, *Acetobacter aceti*, *Acetobacter pasteurianum*, and torula yeast.

If all of this scientific nomenclature inspires you to find out which strains of bacteria and yeast are present in your kombucha culture, you're in luck. The Happy Herbalist website (see Resources, page 79) offers a link to a laboratory that analyzes kombucha cultures.

Acids, Enzymes, and Vitamins

The microorganisms in a kombucha culture produce a number of useful substances, including acids, enzymes, and vitamins, especially B vitamins. Although not all batches of kombucha tea contain the same acids, enzymes, and vitamins, the most commonly reported components are listed here, in alphabetical order:

- acetic acid
- amino acids: alanine, aspartic acid, glutamic acid, isoleucine, leucine, lysine, phenylalanine, serine, threonine, tyrosine, and valine
- carbonic acid
- cobalamin and cyanocobalamin (vitamin B_{12})
- enzymes (various)
- folic acid
- gluconic, glucuronic, and glucaric acid (see page 30)
- lactic acid (see page 29)
- niacin and niacinamide (vitamin B_3)
- pyridoxine (vitamin B_6)
- riboflavin (vitamin B_2)
- thiamine (vitamin B_1)
- usnic acid (Note: Some experts claim that this lichen acid is found in kombucha, but author, botanist, and clinical herbalist Christopher Hobbs claims otherwise.)
- other potential acids: citric acid, hydroxy acid, malonic acid, oxalic acid, succinic acid, and tartaric acid

And there's more. According to Hobbs, many other compounds may be present, contributing to the characteristic sweet-and-sour taste and smell of kombucha tea. These include acetoin; anisaldehyde; diacetyl; isobutyraldehyde; methyl isobutyl ketone; valeraldehyde; vanillic acid; and esters of ethyl, isobutyl, isoamyl alcohols and methyl.

Acid, Alkaline, and Neutral pH

Günther Frank reports that acids have a preservative effect because certain microbes, especially those that create toxins, are unable to tolerate their low pH. To a certain extent, kombucha tea, which is naturally acidic, protects itself from dangerous microbes.

Let's briefly explore the meaning of pH, which is the measure of acidity or alkalinity that's so extremely vital to life. Depicted by a set of numerical values, a solution's pH is measured on a logarithmic scale of zero to 14. The lower the pH, the more acidic the solution, and the higher the pH, the more alkaline the solution. When a solution is neither acid nor alkaline, it has a pH of 7, which is neutral. Kombucha tea is acidic, and its pH varies from 2.8 to 4. When it tastes like cider, kombucha tea has a pH of about 3.

In the human body, pH balance is critical to the maintenance of overall health and survival. Different body fluids have different pH levels. For example, to aid digestion, the pH of the stomach's gastric juices is normally quite acidic, between 1 and 5, while the pH of blood plasma is quite alkaline, falling in the narrow range between 7.35 and 7.45. In healthy people, body fluids maintain their respective pH equilibrium primarily because of the respiratory and urinary systems' regulatory functions, although additional buffering processes help as well.

"Acidosis" describes a state of excessive acidity in body fluids and "alkalosis" excessive alkalinity: neither of these states is desirable. Some researchers say that pH readings tend to increase with age, as the blood becomes more alkaline. Even a slight increase in pH results in lower oxygen levels in the blood and cells. Thus any elevation in pH, no matter how small, indicates the beginning of disease and affects how we age. However, through the buffering process mentioned above, the body keeps pH in strict equilibrium either by liberating hydrogen ions (called protons) to increase acidity or by calling on calcium reserves to increase alkalinity.

If autonomous systems balance our pH levels for us, do we really need to concern ourselves with our pH at any age? Natural healers tell us that acidic foods (such as some fruits) increase alkalinity and alkaline foods (such as milk and bananas) increase acidity. To some extent, you can control your body's pH with your dietary choices. If, for instance, you suffer from an upset stomach due to hyperacidity, you may benefit from eating a sour fruit, such as a sour apple. Although this may seem counterintuitive, relief is almost instantaneous, just as it would be if you chose an alkaline substance, such as a glass of milk, instead. However, when you choose the sour fruit, the potential long-term benefit is greater because you're healing the underlying imbalance rather than temporarily masking the upset.

Because it's acidic, kombucha tea is particularly effective in balancing the body's pH. This raises some interesting questions. For example, can drinking kombucha tea over the long term lower the body's pH, resulting in a kind of rejuvenation? We don't yet have a scientific answer to this question. In the meantime, however, you can test the pH in your saliva and urine by purchasing pH tests at your local pharmacy or on the Internet. The ideal blood pH is 7.35, and saliva pH should fall between 6.4 and 6.8, because saliva is usually more acidic than blood. Urinary pH should fall between 6 and 7, with the results being higher in the evening. If you're new to kombucha tea, why not test your pH values now, then test them again after regularly drinking the tea?

Lactic Acid

Lactic acid fermentation is a process used to make and naturally preserve certain foods and beverages. Some researchers say that some kombucha cultures contain lactic acid, while others claim that no kombucha cultures contain lactic acid. Given the possibility that lactic acid is present in some kombucha cultures, let's explore the topic briefly.

In the lactic acid fermentation process, friendly bacteria, including *Lactobacillus acidophilus* and *Lactobacillus bulgaricus,* are used to make yogurt, kefir, and other cultured milk products. Unlike alcohol fermentation, lactic acid fermentation is a living process that doesn't kill the hardworking microbes. In fact, lactic acid fermentation always creates new bacteria.

FAQ

Q: What is lactic acid fermentation?

A: Lactic acid fermentation is a form of food preservation. Lactic acid is an end product when a carbohydrate, such as sugar, is mixed with friendly microorganisms and allowed to ferment. In kombucha tea, these microorganisms produce mainly L(+) lactic acid, the good acid. The breakdown of glycogen (glycolysis) causes lactic acid to accumulate in active muscle tissues. As discussed in this book, some researchers say that lactic acid shouldn't be found in kombucha tea and that its presence indicates a deterioration of the kombucha culture. Others disagree.

There are two kinds of lactic acids: the "good," or L(+), lactic acid and the "bad," or D(-), lactic acid. Blood, muscle tissue, and the stomach contain the good lactic acid, which improves blood circulation and prevents constipation and decay in the bowels by promoting bowel movements. It also helps to maintain pH balance. In addition, because it's rich in vitamin C, good lactic acid supports the body's natural resistance against infections. It also supports pancreatic function, which in turn stimulates the secretion activity of all the digestive organs.

Bad lactic acid enters the body either through food intake or overexertion of the muscles. Cancer cells contain bad lactic acid that's produced due to lack of oxygen. Bacteria also produce bad lactic acid.

Fermented foods contain both kinds of lactic acid, but usually more of the good lactic acid. According to some sources, kombucha produces primarily good lactic acid. Johannes Kuhl, a German doctor and cancer authority, says kombucha tea, if taken regularly, can prevent chronic conditions from developing. In people who are already ill, the tea also can be used to heal specific ailments.

Gluconic, Glucuronic, and Glucaric Acids

Gluconic acid is important because it helps the body use metallic minerals, such as calcium. Gluconic acid is a byproduct of kombucha fermentation that results from the incomplete oxidation of glucose (sugar). Kombucha experts seem to agree about this fact; however, when it comes to glucuronic and glucaric acids, opinion is split about whether these acids can be found in the kombucha at all.

According to author Betsy Pryor and Pronatura, a company started by Peter Theiss that distributes kombucha products, glucuronic acid is present in the kombucha. However, author and botanist Christopher Hobbs and Kefiplant's Sergi Rollan make counterclaims. Though some researchers report large quantities of glucuronic acid in kombucha tea, Hobbs says this is impossible and no credible laboratory analysis of kombucha tea has found glucuronic acid. According to Rollan, glucuronic acid, if present in kombucha, indicates spoilage. Despite this controversy, let's examine glucuronic acid in more detail.

Glucuronic acid is a compound used by the liver for detoxification. It's an important metabolite that the healthy liver produces. The glucuronic acid binds with metabolic and environmental toxins and poisons, which are then excreted. Once toxins are bound to glucuronic acid, the body can't reabsorb them. According to Günther Frank, this detoxification process is responsible for healing gout, rheumatism, and arthritis because the offending toxins are flushed out through the urine in the bound-up form of glucuronides, or conjugated glucuronic acids. Glucuronic acid may also play an important role in preventing wrinkling of the skin. The presence of glucuronic acid could account for the broad range of health benefits enjoyed by those who drink kombucha tea.

Older research that dates back to the 1970s and 1980s involved the chemical analysis of kombucha tea and suggested that glucuronic acid was a key component. The idea that glucuronic acid is present in kombucha was based on the observation that glucuronic acid conjugates in urine increase after consumption of kombucha tea. These analyses were done using gas chromatography, which identifies different chemical compounds and is a method that relies on having proper chemical standards to match to unknown chemicals. According to Pronatura, Rudolf Sklenar's formula for kombucha tea contained glucuronic acid. In addition, Betsy Pryor has asserted that both the

Kombucha: The Acid Controversy

Not all kombucha experts agree about exactly which acids can be found in a kombucha culture. For example, the professionals from Kefiplant (see chapter 6) say that a high-quality kombucha culture shouldn't contain lactic acid other than in negligible trace amounts. They believe that a kombucha culture will produce lactic acid only if it has mutated. Furthermore, they claim that kombucha shouldn't contain glucuronic acid and that any kombucha that contains glucuronic acid will also contain toxic molecules and should be avoided.

US Food and Drug Administration and the state of California confirmed that properly prepared kombucha tea contained glucuronic acid.

More recent and thorough analyses of a variety of commercial and home-brewed versions of kombucha tea have found no evidence of glucuronic acid. Rather, these analyses suggest that glucaric acid, which helps eliminate the conjugated glucuronic acid produced by the liver, is present. Thus, the new claim goes, glucaric acid probably makes the liver more efficient. In addition, glucaric acid, which is found in fruits and vegetables, is being explored as a cancer-preventive agent.

Perhaps the most useful perspective is to recognize that these acids support a healthy liver. If you have a history of smoking, using commercial antibiotics or other pharmaceuticals, drug addiction, alcohol abuse, or eating excessive amounts of junk food, your overtaxed liver could use help. Kombucha tea seems to contain key elements that accelerate detoxification. Combine kombucha tea drinking with milk thistle liver treatment, and you may feel rejuvenated even more quickly.

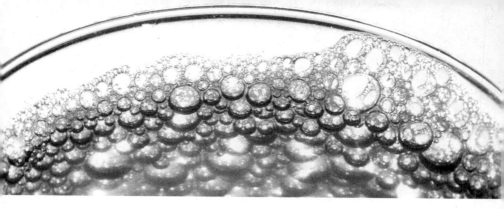

Chapter Four
Health Benefits

No ironclad scientific research results currently exist to confirm the health benefits of drinking kombucha tea. For now we can only say that the benefits are as real as the personal testimonials—and there are many—that praise the tea's effects. We must also realize that the tea, like any other remedy, might not work for everyone.

Drinking kombucha tea can be most effective in supporting overall wellness and vitality when it's done in conjunction with other healthful practices. No one can continually make poor choices that endanger his or her health and get away with it simply by sipping a little kombucha tea once or twice a day. Germans are fond of quoting a proverb that embodies this idea: "The jug continues going to the fountain until it breaks." As long as we take good care of our jug—our body—it will last a long time. If we abuse it, it will break prematurely.

Before looking more closely at the many health benefits of kombucha tea, we must realize that kombucha isn't a magic potion. Author and botanist Christopher Hobbs, for one, has warned kombucha users against expecting a miracle. Contrary to the promise that appears in the "Manchurian" leaflet depicted in the introduction (see page 3), kombucha tea isn't a source of immortality.

But let's examine the other side of the coin. Kombucha tea does seem like a cure-all because throughout its long history, many people have reported that the tea restored their health and alleviated ailments of various kinds. Such testimonials clearly and overwhelmingly support the hypothesis that kombucha tea wondrously restores the body.

Kombucha expert and author Betsy Pryor confesses that she was once a nonbeliever. But her research and personal experience with kombucha made her a convert, and she went on to share her knowledge and faith in kombucha tea through her books and lectures. During a seminar, she volunteered her initial impressions about kombucha tea: "I thought it was snake oil. I really want to be honest about that. It did too many things. I didn't think it was possible for any one thing to affect arthritis to T cells to psoriasis. I just didn't believe it."

In time, however, Pryor's cynical view changed. Rudolf Sklenar's impeccable research in Germany and additional research conducted in Russia convinced her that kombucha tea can help the body to heal itself. At the same time, she is the first to admit that kombucha tea "isn't a cure for anything." What she means by this is that kombucha tea doesn't work like a drug. Instead, what it does is boost the body's own abilities to heal itself, making kombucha tea far more powerful, potent, and valuable than any drug could ever be.

If you currently share Betsy Prior's initial impression of kombucha tea, try to keep an open mind. If skeptics like Pryor can be beguiled by kombucha's charms, you might be as well.

As I've mentioned, homeopathic doctors and other practitioners have successfully treated patients using kombucha tea, so I feel the tea can't simply be dismissed as snake oil. In time, scientific tests will confirm what we have seen and experienced—kombucha tea can work miracles.

Kombucha Tea Regimen and Dosage

I have heard from regular users of kombucha tea that their enjoyment of living increases the longer they drink the tea. Many tell me they've resumed activities for which they previously had lost the energy. While I'm always happy to hear about these positive results, I recommend against using any supplement or remedy on a regular basis over long periods. There's evidence that the effect of any remedy diminishes if it's continued without a break. That's why experienced healers recommend a regimen that has an off-and-on pattern, which is more consistent with the natural rhythm of life.

How you design your kombucha tea regimen is up to you. For instance, you might find that a pattern of five days on and two days off works for you. Or you could try five weeks on and two weeks off or five months on and two months off. Choose what suits your needs and lifestyle. When you're particularly stressed or ill, you may want to continue drinking the tea for a longer period until you feel well again and are ready for another break in the pattern.

I've been asked, "Can I drink too much kombucha tea?" While this is a question for your health care practitioner, I'm happy to describe my own routine. My wife and I drink ½ cup (120 milliliters) of kombucha tea on an empty stomach early in the morning and another ½ cup before going to bed at night. We're planning to increase our intake to 1 cup (8 ounces or about 240 milliliters) in the morning and 1 cup in the evening. However, this is a dosage that we have decided is right for us and not a general recommendation for others.

The answer to the dosage question varies depending on the expert being consulted. Recommendations vary from ½ cup on an empty stomach to ¼ cup (60 milliliters) before each meal to ½ cup after the main meal of the day. I would suggest that the amount and timing aren't critical, provided you regularly drink reasonable amounts of kombucha tea when you're not taking a break from it as part of your "off-and-on" cycle.

I have also been asked, "What is the suggested amount for children?" I'm not aware of one specific recommendation. The response depends on the age of the child and personal preference. Common sense says to decrease the amount by as much as 80 percent or as little as 20 percent, depending on the child's age and size.

Kombucha Tea and Unwanted Side Effects

If the kombucha and the fermentation process are properly handled, most people shouldn't experience any unwanted side effects after drinking kombucha tea. Diabetics are one possible exception; if you have diabetes, you may want to take the additional precaution of carefully monitoring the tea's sugar content.

For the most part, if you follow the recommendations in this book, you shouldn't have any problems, but let's consider what some kombucha experts have to say. Harald Tietze reportedly drank up to three quarts (three liters) of kombucha tea every day for six weeks and felt great. (I'm not recommending this; start slowly if you plan to use the tea, and note typical dosages, page 35.) Tietze would probably be very confident in stating that the tea has no unwanted side effects. Christopher Hobbs, however, quotes a mushroom cultivator in the state of Washington who is strongly opposed to the use of kombucha tea because he fears the culture could be contaminated by pathogenic microbes. Is it possible? I'm not aware of any literature that supports this fear.

Betsy Pryor reports that both the US Food and Drug Administration and the State of California frequently inspected batches of her kombucha tea and found them to be completely safe. Remember, the kombucha culture has the natural ability to protect itself against harmful bacteria. Even Hobbs agrees that with proper and careful preparation, kombucha tea should be safe. And millions of people all around the world seem to safely drink kombucha tea and consume other fermented drinks and foods.

Ultimately, it's up to you to decide whether or not you feel comfortable using kombucha tea. I have shared relevant information from private and professional sources, but you must evaluate the evidence to determine whether or not you deem kombucha tea to be appropriate for your needs.

Kombucha Tea and Cancer

I believe that cancer is a systemic disease that requires holistic treatment, and approaches that combine various remedies simultaneously may work best. Kombucha tea has been found to play a supportive role in cancer therapy. As discussed in chapter 2, German medical doctor Rudolf Sklenar used kombucha tea extensively to treat cancer patients. Despite this fact, some credible researchers say there's no clinical evidence to support the role of kombucha tea in cancer therapy. Sklenar used kombucha tea to treat cancer because he was familiar with lactic acid fermentation and its role in prevention and healing. In the Canadian edition of *How to Fight Cancer & Win,* a chapter titled "The Healing Power of Lactic Acid" explains how lactic acid works to repress cancer cells without harming healthy cells.

Author Rosina Fasching says kombucha tea can fight cancer because of its ability to restore the human body's metabolism to the energetic, natural state that healthy, active people of all ages enjoy. Offering a possible explanation of how kombucha tea overcomes cancer, Fasching says the kombucha fungus sprouts in an acidic environment that eliminates or retards the development of primitive cancer-causing microbes that thrive in alkaline environments. Indicating that the cancer-causing microbe is a fungus, Fasching says the key to treating cancer is simple: fungus versus fungus.

We know that intestinal flora, the friendly bacteria in our gut, play an important role in displacing and destroying carcinogens, and perhaps even cancer-causing microbes. Researcher Günther Enderlein says kombucha's positive microbial action has the power to destroy the carcinogenic terrain that enables cancer to grow. By cleansing the system, restoring the intestinal flora, and balancing the body's crucial pH, kombucha helps the immune system regain control over proliferating cancer cells. Furthermore, Enderlein says that a cancer-enhancing microbe is the culprit responsible for causing cancer cells to divide unnaturally and unchecked. He states that only natural methods, such as drinking kombucha tea, can effectively fight cancer.

I happen to agree with Enderlein. There's overwhelming evidence that orthodox cancer therapies are failing. I saw my own mother destroyed by cancer over a ten-year period, even as she submitted to surgery, radiation, and chemotherapy. These treatment methods are still standard today, and orthodox medicine continues to devise new and more aggressive ways of employing intensive chemotherapy.

We know that some famous figures have used kombucha tea and overcome cancer. For example, Ronald Reagan, former president of the United States, was diagnosed with cancer while he was in office. His treatment became public knowledge and was discussed widely in the media. Reportedly, Reagan obtained a kombucha culture from Japan and drank about one quart (one liter) of the tea daily. Reagan's cancer was prevented from spreading, and he ultimately died of the effects of Alzheimer's disease, which suggests that he may have been freed of cancer.

Kombucha researcher Günther Frank said at the time that Reagan got news of the cancer-fighting powers of kombucha tea from Aleksandr Solzhenitsyn, author and Nobel Prize winner, who was diagnosed with cancer in 1952. According to his book *The Cancer Ward,* Solzhenitsyn conquered cancer in 1953 in a hospital in Tashkent, Russia. Solzhenitsyn also reported that when he was exiled in a prison colony in Siberia, he and others survived mainly due to the kombucha tea they fermented and drank.

Kombucha Tea for Diabetics

Some experts recommend that people with diabetes avoid kombucha tea because of the tea's potential sugar content. As discussed in previous chapters, there should be little concern about preparing kombucha tea with white sugar, however, because the sugar is almost completely used up by the bacteria and yeast during fermentation. Nonetheless, a Viennese professor prepared a sugarless kombucha tea in the 1920s. The tea was tested on people with diabetes. In some subjects, test results showed a noticeable lowering of blood sugar levels. Many other subjects reported improvement in their overall well-being. The researcher ascribed the effect to the gluconic acid present in the tea. At that time, medical practitioners held gluconic acid in high regard because, unlike glucose or dextrose, it was thought that people with diabetes could burn the gluconic acid and use its high energy content.

While this research is intriguing, according to Kefiplant's Sergi Rollan, there can be no such thing as "sugarless" kombucha tea because it's impossible to create kombucha tea without sugar. Some commercial kombucha products contain less sugar than home-brewed kombucha teas, so these drinks may be more suitable for diabetics. However, when home brews are left to ferment for a few extra days, all of the sugar is used up in fermentation, resulting in a vinegary and essentially sugar-free drink.

The Key Ingredients

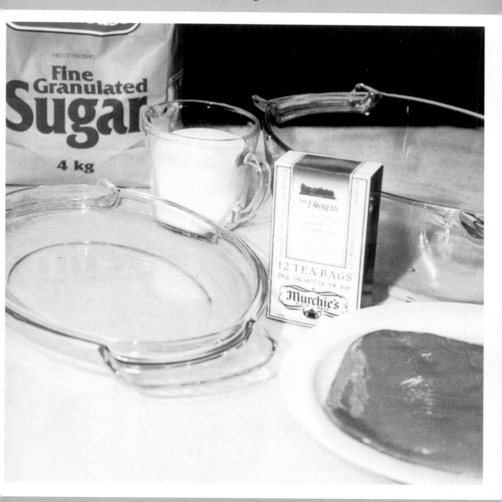

Ingredients and Tools

- Kombucha Mushroom
- Orange Pekoe Tea
- Refined White Sugar
- Purified Water
- Funnel
- Stainless Steel Pot

- Large Glass Bowl or Dish
- Glass Storage Containers
- Wooden or Ceramic Spoon
- White Cotton Towel or Cheesecloth

The tea ceremony: Making the tea and sugar solution

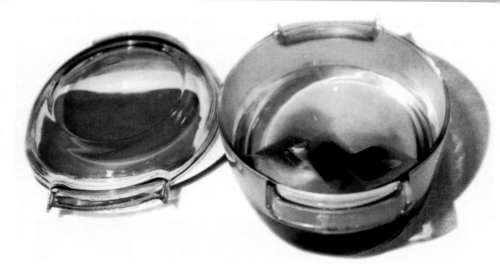

Let the tea cool to lukewarm before adding your kombucha mushroom.

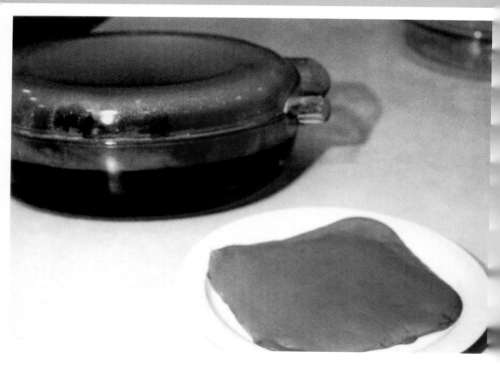

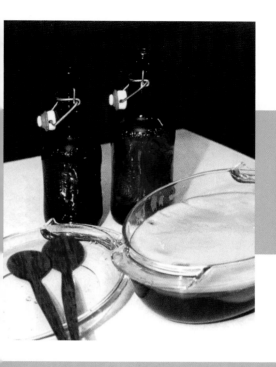

The fermenting process: The mushroom converts the sugar and tea into a variety of enzymes, acids and vitamins.

Take a look at your baby kombucha.

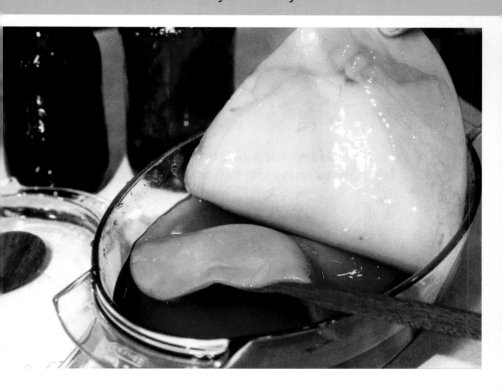

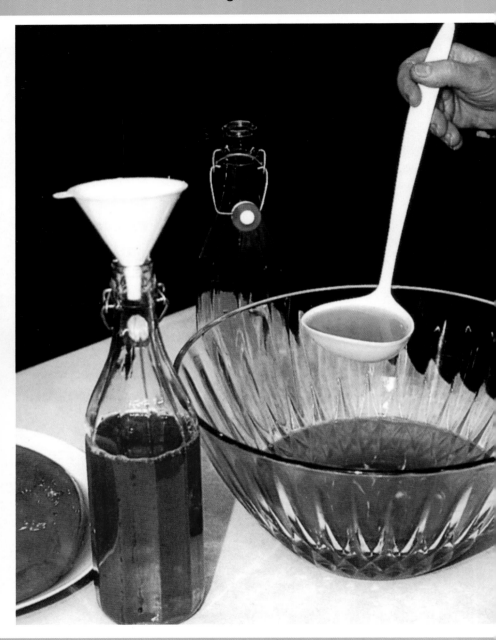

It's time to enjoy the delicious, healing drink.

There's a story that Joseph Stalin, former leader of the Soviet Union, was paranoid about contracting cancer and encouraged research into possible cancer cures. His researchers found a region in Russia (Solikamsk and Berezniki) that was practically void of cancer occurrences, with only a few cases reported among immigrants. Eventually the researchers came across the region's popular tea kvass, and subsequent investigation by the Central Bacteriological Institute in Moscow found the tea kvass to be none other than kombucha tea formed by the symbiotic growths of *Acetobacter xylinum* and yeast cells of the genus *Saccharomyces*. There's no evidence that the discovery aided Stalin, however, because KGB (Soviet State Security Committee) agents reportedly convinced him to have his physician jailed.

Kombucha Tea and Specific Health Conditions

Following is an overview of the primary health effects reported for kombucha tea. Drinking kombucha tea seems to alleviate a number of ailments. In addition, it helps to prevent the onset of illness and promote health even as we age. Note: Seeking the advice of a holistic health practitioner before using kombucha tea to treat any condition is recommended.

AIDS (acquired immune deficiency syndrome). AIDS, a highly publicized ailment, is a syndrome, rather than a single disease, that impairs the immune system. It's caused by exposure to HIV, a retrovirus that infects helper T cells and other vital cells in the immune system. I worked with AIDS patients during drug trials at St. Paul's Hospital in Vancouver, British Columbia, in the early years. In 1991, we knew that once the disease is active, there isn't a cure. Despite treatment, AIDS victims died within two years of disease manifestation. By 1995, medical science had extended this to three years. Now, decades later, newer drugs have the potential to prolong the lifespan of people with AIDS by many years. In fact, HIV-infected patients on a modern drug regimen can nowadays apparently look forward to a normal lifespan, provided the HIV condition is not allowed to deteriorate to AIDS.

According to Betsy Pryor, kombucha tea can help boost immunity and keep the virus contained for a longer period. This use of kombucha tea is currently under study. Note: Caution is advisable before patients experiment on their own with any homemade remedies that promise better T-cell counts. Some authors warn people with AIDS or HIV against using kombucha tea and advise that further research is necessary.

Arthritis. Individuals with arthritis have reported healing effects from drinking kombucha tea. Many dancers, both in Russia and North America, drink kombucha tea and report fewer ligament and arthritis problems, both of which are common among dancers and other athletes.

Asthma. According to author Harald Tietze, asthma patients under the care of a physician named A. Wiesner noticed considerable improvement in their condition while on kombucha therapy.

Blood pressure, high. High blood pressure is a persistent health problem that has many causes, although it's often closely associated with high blood cholesterol levels. Just as there are many causes, there are many treatments. Drinking kombucha tea regularly has been known to lower high blood pressure. In addition, I would recommend adding nutrient silica gel to the daily diet to elasticize the blood vessels. And, of course, avoid salt!

Bowel problems. Kombucha tea can help heal so many illnesses of the stomach and the bowels that I could write a whole book on this subject alone. Kombucha tea shows good results in clearing up stomach and bowel problems by balancing the pH and the intestinal flora. Healing seems to follow magically once the body's systems are in good working order.

Bronchitis. According to Harald Tietze, a Dutch doctor by the name of Harnisch successfully prescribed kombucha tea for treating bronchitis in his young patients.

***Candida albicans* infection.** Because *Candida albicans* is a type of yeast infection, it's natural to assume that people who have it should stay away from other yeast cultures. On the contrary, Günther Frank says the yeast in the kombucha culture doesn't belong to the *Candida* family. He argues that this is precisely why it can help fight off the troublesome *Candida albicans* infections that plague so many people, especially women. Frank goes on to explain that *Candida* yeast reproduces by means of spores, whereas other types of yeast reproduce by means of budding (or a combination of budding and fission) and don't have spores. The yeast in the kombucha culture reproduces by fission. Frank's argument is supported by studies done at Cornell University and reported by Betsy Pryor. The Cornell studies found kombucha tea effective in treating *Candida albicans* and the bacteria that commonly cause duodenal ulcers.

I recently heard a fifty-year-old tax accountant with a yeast infection give a testimonial about kombucha tea in Las Vegas. She said she was spending about $30 a month on prescription drugs. Three weeks after starting to drink kombucha tea, she stopped taking the drugs and hasn't used them since. Her *Candida* problems have disappeared.

Note: Drinking kombucha tea as a remedy for *Candida* isn't advisable without guidance from a naturopath.

Cholesterol levels, high. We all know that high blood lipid levels (excessive cholesterol) and hypertension (high blood pressure) ultimately lead to cardiovascular disease, the number one killer in North America. Drinking kombucha tea has been found to decrease blood cholesterol levels.

Chronic fatigue syndrome. Many researchers have reported that people attribute drinking kombucha tea to healing chronic fatigue syndrome. If chronic fatigue is due to intestinal or liver problems, as some people believe, kombucha tea, with its cleansing and balancing abilities, could be a key factor in preventing and overcoming this syndrome.

Colds. Cold viruses take hold of us mainly when we're stressed, tired, or depressed or when the immune system is compromised. Because kombucha functions as a natural antibiotic, regularly drinking kombucha tea can help prevent or alleviate colds. Adding vitamin C to a cold prevention program is vital. Some holistic healers also recommend echinacea for cold prevention. KefiActive (see page 73) offers two products that are designed to fight colds:

KefiActive Astragalus Membranaceus Root, which combats frequent colds, and KefiActive Echinacea, which fights off upper respiratory tract infections.

Constipation. Constipation is often chronic and caused by eating the wrong foods or getting insufficient exercise. Much like diarrhea, constipation has reportedly been cleared up quickly by kombucha tea. Perhaps that's because drinking kombucha tea helps to restore intestinal flora.

In addition to drinking kombucha tea, another good habit that prevents constipation is eating a sufficient daily amount of fiber-rich food, or roughage. Eating foods such as green salads, fruits, and whole-grain breads becomes even more important with age, because digestion tends to become more sluggish and needs all the encouragement it can get. Roughage and kombucha tea are excellent natural laxatives, and if you're incorporating both into your diet, you won't be likely to develop constipation. According to experts, even the classic prune juice remedy shouldn't be needed when drinking kombucha tea.

Diarrhea. Kombucha tea seems to clear up diarrhea quickly. Scientific studies in Russia indicate that bacterial dysentery also responds well to kombucha tea.

Fluid retention. Testimonials support findings that drinking kombucha tea can reduce excessive fluid retention in the legs.

Gout. Gout can result when a person eats too much rich food over many years. Because kombucha tea balances the intestinal flora and stimulates metabolism, drinking the tea could be a helpful remedy for gout. Juice fasting that incorporates kombucha tea could also help alleviate gout.

Immunity. Because drinking kombucha tea energizes and boosts metabolism, it automatically fosters the health of the immune system. In addition, I suggest taking additional steps to heal an impaired immune system. These steps include adopting a holistic lifestyle, eating a healthful diet, and sticking to an ongoing detoxification program. Such actions are particularly important in the case of severe impairment, such as liver poisoning or HIV infection. Other diseases, including cancer, also may be easier to overcome when the immune system is operating at full capacity. Of course, we would all like to have a superbly functioning immune response. Drinking kombucha tea seems to be a valuable move in that direction.

Impotence. In kombucha tea, we have a panacea for impotence. Potency depends on vitality, which the tea can support. (Drinking the tea wouldn't be effective, however, in cases involving a physical or severe mental disability.) In addition, Rudolf Sklenar and others have reported that kombucha tea can have a toning effect on the male sex organs.

Kidney problems. Among other therapies, drinking adequate amounts of healthful liquids is necessary to flush the kidneys and keep them in top shape. Drinking kombucha tea could aid kidney flushing. According to Harald Tietze, comparison trials conducted by a physician named A. Wiesner resulted in an 89 percent success rate of kombucha over an interferon drug.

Kidney stones. People who don't drink enough fluids are generally more prone to developing kidney stones. For this reason, simply drinking tea is beneficial because tea drinkers have increased fluid intake. In addition, studies have shown that drinking kombucha tea helps dissolve the stones.

Multiple sclerosis. Betsy Pryor reports impressive testimonial evidence that kombucha tea heals multiple sclerosis. In addition, Harald Tietze says that a woman from Holland claims she was healed by drinking kombucha tea. According to a letter published in the Dutch magazine *Op Zoek,* the woman started drinking kombucha tea and in less than one year she was no longer tired and even got her driver's license back. She also said she planned to go skiing again. Of course, clinical studies are needed to confirm whether this encouraging experience can be replicated among others with multiple sclerosis.

Prostate problems. Extremely common in older men, prostate problems are thought to affect half of men over age fifty. Many natural remedies are available. Alternative health experts suggest that drinking kombucha tea regularly decreases bladder inflammation and can therefore alleviate prostate

FAQ

Q: Can kombucha tea cure cancer?

A: No one can be sure whether or not kombucha tea cures cancer, but some physicians have reduced tumors by prescribing nothing other than kombucha tea. Notably, these practitioners include Rudolf Sklenar and Johannes Kuhl.

Q: Is kombucha tea a miracle cure?

A: Kombucha tea isn't a cure for any disease. Rather, the tea is best used as part of a health-supporting regimen that includes optimal nutrition, exercise, rest, and last but not least, spiritual nourishment. Kombucha tea aids digestion, improves metabolism, and provides extra energy. For these reasons, it can be a benefit to anyone who is suffering from deficient health. If you have been diagnosed with a serious disease, you should consult your health care practitioner before trying kombucha tea.

Q: Can I eat the kombucha culture?

A: While eating a kombucha culture is possible, it's not recommended. My advice is to keep the kombucha alive to make more batches of healthful tea. The kombucha culture contains the same components as the tea, only in concentrated form. Apparently some people have eaten it and benefited, but why bother? The condensed form contains cellulose that the human body can't metabolize, and it probably doesn't taste pleasant. For those who are interested in additional sources of kombucha, commercial kombucha extracts are sold in natural food stores, mainly for use by people who have diabetes.

inflammation too. Other natural remedies include hemp oil, organic nettle root, pomegranate seeds, pumpkin seeds, willow, and zinc supplements.

When it comes to prostate cancer, even orthodox medicine is increasingly recognizing that invasive therapies or surgery may not always be the best answer. A panel of doctors suggested that men should no longer get routine prostate-specific antigen (PSA) tests. As reported in the *New York Times* in October 2011, the rationale for discouraging men from having PSA tests is based on the fact that men suffering from extremely slow-growing prostate cancer die of other causes before the prostate cancer becomes life threatening.

Psoriasis. Some medical practitioners reportedly recommend kombucha tea for psoriasis. In addition to drinking the tea, those with psoriasis can apply the tea directly to the skin. Testimonials tend to confirm this. Adding nutrient silica gel to the diet is another good way to clear up and prevent skin disease, especially for people who are genetically predisposed to it. Stress also seems to play a role in triggering skin rashes. In such cases, removing the source of the stress while increasing the intake of B-complex vitamins can be helpful.

Rheumatism. Harald Tietze writes that a physician named A. Wiesner reported a 92 percent success rate using kombucha tea to treat trial subjects with rheumatism. The subjects' pain diminished and they were able to move limbs freely.

Sleep disorders. Despite established guidelines for sleep requirements by age (babies need about sixteen hours per day, and older adults need around seven hours), sleep is highly individual and therefore variable. Sometimes I need twelve hours of sleep and other times I need only three. For a person who has no underlying ailments, drinking a glass of kombucha tea just before bedtime can help overcome problems with falling asleep and not sleeping soundly.

Stomach problems. See "bowel problems," page 40.

Tonsillitis. Russian researchers have reported that kombucha tea can reduce the inflammation of tonsillitis. In my opinion, tonsils should be removed surgically only in the direst circumstances. My own naturopathic family doctor saved me from tonsillectomy, and I have always credited my resistance to infections and colds to my protective tonsils fighting off intruders.

Doggone Good for Animals

Many people give kombucha tea to their dogs and cats to drink to improve their health. According to some experts, including Betsy Pryor, the tea eliminates doggie breath and extreme body odor. Scientific research involving other animals also has had promising outcomes. The former Soviet Union embarked on extensive research on kombucha in veterinary use. A preparation made from the kombucha symbiosis was tried on sheep, cows, and other mammals. In clinical trials, young sheep and cows with dysentery and colibacillosis were given the kombucha preparation, resulting in a 100 percent recovery rate. In addition, mixing the kombucha preparation into chicken feed led to a 15 percent increase in the growth rate of baby chicks.

FAQ

Q: Can I give kombucha tea to my pet?

A: Yes, kombucha tea can be given safely to your furry loved ones. One tablespoon per day is sufficient for many pets; however, larger animals can be given twice that dosage. Simply add the tea to the pet's drinking water or food or use a small syringe to administer the tea orally.

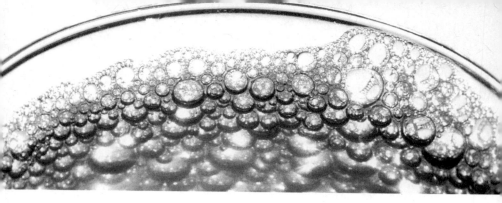

Chapter Five
Making Kombucha Tea

Why make your own kombucha tea? Simply because it's one of the greatest hobbies you can have and a fun activity you can share with your loved ones. Your hobby will provide you with a health-supporting beverage that's delicious, inexpensive, and free of preservatives. Making kombucha tea can also be a truly altruistic act if you pass along the brew and kombucha babies to others.

Many cultures, especially those in Asia and Europe, have established certain rituals that involve the making and presentation of tea. In any successful tea ceremony, time is a critical factor. "Never rush a tea ceremony," my mother told me ages ago. How much time does it take to make kombucha tea? After you've gotten the hang of it, it takes about thirty minutes to brew and some additional time to cool. Then, of course, you must wait several days while the tea ferments. Be patient and go slowly if this is your first experience making the tea. The time you spend reading these instructions, especially the preliminary information about ingredients and equipment, will be a valuable investment.

Get to Know the Ingredients

You need only four items to make kombucha tea. The first is the kombucha culture. The remaining ingredients—tea, white sugar, and purified water—are probably already in your kitchen.

The Kombucha Culture

The most important ingredient in kombucha tea, of course, is the kombucha! So where can you get your very own kombucha baby? Perhaps a relative, friend, or neighbor has already offered one to you. If not, see Resources (page 79) for information about where to obtain a kombucha starter kit.

In all likelihood, your first kombucha will reach you in a sealed plastic bag, and it will be floating in a small amount of nourishing kombucha tea. You'll notice that the culture looks like a pancake: flat and golden brown. Touch it, however, and you'll find that it doesn't feel like most pancakes; the kombucha should feel rubbery and slightly oily.

Cleanliness is essential for handling your kombucha baby. So before you touch it, make sure your hands are clean. Wash your hands with soap and warm water and rinse all of the soapy residue off your fingers. Wearing clean rubber gloves is an option, though I prefer being in direct contact with the kombucha. While cleanliness is important, sterile conditions aren't necessary since intruding organisms will be destroyed during fermentation.

The kombucha culture must be protected from contact with certain items. For example, the kombucha can leach toxins from metal, so you must remove all rings and jewelry from fingers and wrists before touching it. You must also avoid using equipment that's metal or may contain metal during certain stages of the process. Similarly, avoid using plastic equipment and utensils because the kombucha can draw out harmful chemicals that are in plastics. Finally, the kombucha culture may be damaged or even die if it's exposed to tobacco smoke. The following sections provide important details you need to know about these precautions and sensitivities.

No Metal, No Plastic

The kombucha culture can't tolerate contact with any kind of metal, so it's necessary to avoid bowls and other pieces of equipment that are made of metal when making kombucha tea. The kombucha can leach metal from bowls and various kitchen tools.

I recommend that only glass bowls and containers be used for fermenting and storing kombucha tea. Avoid crystal bowls. Since crystal contains lead, there's a danger that the kombucha culture will absorb the lead from the crystal. Lead is highly poisonous, not only to the kombucha but also to humans. Ceramic and porcelain bowls present a similar problem since they contain metallic elements.

Plastic containers should never be used for fermenting kombucha tea. The kombucha culture has the power to leach dangerous compounds from plastic as well as metal. I've seen plenty of information in the media that drives home the dangers of estrogenic compounds in ordinary plastic containers that we use every day, especially in our kitchens, and how they endanger us and the environment. Because these estrogenic compounds in plastics so closely mimic the female hormone estrogen, they're creating havoc among the males of many species. For example, there has been an increase in the number of boys being born with poorly developed sex organs and a simultaneous rise in hermaphroditic, or intersex, births. Similar aberrations have occurred in animals, especially in fish and other water species that are exposed to concentrated toxins and oil spills (oil is a primary component in plastics).

So if we can't use metal, crystal, ceramic, porcelain, or plastic, we have only one safe alternative for fermenting and storing kombucha tea: unadulterated glass made of the white sands of silica. A large Pyrex glass bowl is the best container to use when fermenting the tea. Remember, however, that while Pyrex bowls are safe to use in the oven, they can't be used to boil water on the stovetop. A friend of mine did this recently. When he had finished brewing the tea, he heard his daughter cry out, "Papa! Papa! Come quickly, your kombucha!" In the kitchen, he found his glass bowl broken and his tea all over the stove and dripping onto the floor. The bowl had shattered in reaction to the heat. The moral of this story: Never heat a Pyrex glass container on the stovetop. Instead, use a stainless steel pot to heat the water for your kombucha tea. This is perfectly safe because the kombucha is never put into the pot.

Just as the tea must be fermented in a glass container, it must also be stored in glass. Thoroughly washed wine bottles that can be corked are the perfect receptacles. The cork allows the tea to breathe, which is important because some fermentation continues even when the tea is stored in the refrigerator.

No Smoking

Experts have reported that tobacco smoke will interfere with the successful fermentation of kombucha tea. In fact, if it's exposed to tobacco smoke during fermentation, the kombucha culture will not prosper and may even die. This isn't surprising when you consider that tobacco is a deadly poison that farmers employ successfully as an insecticide.

In our home, my wife and I don't permit smoking of any tobacco products, which is good for my kombucha cultures. Other noxious fumes, such as automobile exhaust, can also harm the kombucha. For that reason, I wouldn't recommend leaving the tea in your garage to ferment. If your basement opens to the garage, you must find another spot for the fermenting process. Alternatives include the attic, kitchen, or any other area where the culture can be kept warm, undisturbed, and away from direct sunlight. For more recommendations and precautions, see "Choosing the Best Spot for Fermentation," page 61.

The Tea

Tea does more than lend its fantastic flavor to the home-brewed kombucha drink. Tea also provides necessary mineral salts and nitrogen, and it stimulates growth among the bacteria and yeast. When making kombucha tea, you can use black, green, or white tea. I normally use Twinings brand orange pekoe teabags.

No matter which kind of tea you choose, the same general guidelines apply: Use 2 teaspoons of loose tea or 2 tea bags for every quart (liter) of water. The amount can be varied to taste or to make the tea weaker or stronger.

White Tea

White tea, especially organic white tea, has recently become more widely available and is a very popular choice among those who brew kombucha tea. The oldest type of tea from China, white tea comes from the buds and younger leaves of the *Camellia sinensis* plant and gets its name from the silver-white hairs on the unopened buds. Common varieties of white tea include Silvery Tip Pekoe, Silver Needle White Hair, China White, and Fujian White.

White tea contains high levels of catechins, a group of polyphenol antioxidants known to fight free radicals. There are claims that drinking white tea provides protection from a number of ailments, including arterial disease, diabetes, stroke, heart failure, skin damage from ultraviolet radiation, and even cancer and tumor formation. In fact, the polyphenol compounds have been shown to protect against certain types of cancer in scientific studies. The catechins in white tea have also been found to reduce cholesterol, decrease blood pressure, and strengthen blood vessels, thereby reducing the overall risk of cardiovascular disease. Catechins are also believed to have antibacterial and antiviral properties; in scientific testing, they were proven to protect animals from pathogens such as *Salmonella typhimurium*. Finally, the antioxidants in white tea help boost immunity and can be of benefit to humans and animals suffering from compromised immune systems.

Scientific research has confirmed the health benefits of white tea. A 2009 study at Kingston University in London, England, revealed strong anti-inflammatory and antioxidant properties, indicating that the tea could reduce users' risk of developing rheumatoid arthritis, some cancers, and heart disease. Other properties were shown to slow the enzymatic breakdown of elastin and collagen, which naturally accompanies aging. A 1984 study conducted at Pace University in New York showed that white tea extract slows the growth of viruses and bacteria, thereby reducing the incidence of *Staphylococcus* and *Streptococcus* infections as well as pneumonia, fungus growth, and even dental plaque. Additional research at the University Hospitals of Cleveland and Case Western Reserve University revealed that white tea protects skin cells that are exposed to harmful ultraviolet radiation.

It follows that by choosing white tea to make kombucha tea, you're getting not only a brew that tastes great but also one that boasts superior health benefits. Nevertheless, many kombucha enthusiasts still swear they obtain the best results using regular black tea, especially orange pekoe and English breakfast teas.

Caffeine

The amount of caffeine in black, green, or white tea can vary widely. If you're concerned about caffeine content, kombucha tea expert Betsy Pryor assures that the amount of caffeine in the fermented tea is minimal. Just as little or no sugar remains when the tea is harvested, there's almost no caffeine left at the end of the fermentation process.

Some people who are concerned about caffeine might hit on the idea of using herbal tea when making kombucha tea. This might not be such a good idea, as the next section explains.

Herbal Tea

Many kombucha experts recommend against using herbal tea because it contains alkaloids that might affect the kombucha. Others suggest that using teas that contain certain herbs, such as raspberry leaves, blackberry leaves, or dandelions, can enhance kombucha tea. Ideally, the herbal teas should be made from homegrown herbs to ensure they're uncontaminated and as fresh as possible.

I understand why some kombucha hobbyists might want to embark on trials with herbal teas. However, I recommend that they first familiarize themselves with the medicinal effects of the herbal tea they wish to experiment with. This can be accomplished by studying a book about herbs or taking a course from a qualified herbalist. If you gain this expertise and wish to experiment, keep in mind that herbal tea requires only half the amount of steeping time as black tea.

White Sugar

The general guideline for making kombucha tea is to use ½ cup of refined white sugar per quart (liter) of water. The white sugar can be refined from cane or beet sugar.

I know how tough it is to convince health-conscious people that it's okay to use refined white sugar. Keep in mind, however, that the white sugar is in the tea for one reason and one reason alone: to feed the bacteria and yeast cells. The sugar is *not* there to feed *you*. The bacteria and yeast consume the sugar during fermentation. By the time you drink the kombucha tea, there's little, if any, sugar left. Günther Frank has provided a precise example by saying that after a fermentation period of 14 days, only about .1 ounce (3 grams) of simple sugars remains in about 3.5 ounces (100 grams) of kombucha tea. Compare that to the 7 teaspoons (35 grams) of sugar that are present in only one serving of carbonated cola.

White sugar plays many roles during the fermentation of kombucha tea. It assists in the development of organic acids and alcohol, creates new nutrients and vitamins, and helps to transform minerals into the gluconate or acetate forms of organic acids. It also helps develop other new nutrients and polysaccharides.

Still, some kombucha tea brewers continue to experiment with other sweeteners. At one kombucha seminar, an attendee stated, "I reasoned out . . . you should use raw sugar (instead of white refined sugar) because you don't have the elements that you would have in a raw sugar." Then he emphasized, "Which, of course, you find in molasses . . . one of the great foods in the world. So I throw a little molasses into mine, and I find that the rate of reaction from this is approximately three times faster in forming the drink." The lecturer, Betsy Pryor, cautioned the audience against this approach. She said that although certain ingredients, including raw sugar and honey, prompt the kombucha tea to ferment more quickly, research conducted in Russia confirmed that refined white sugar makes the most active type of kombucha tea. If you think you can avoid refined white sugar by using brown sugar, remember that brown sugar, for the most part, is made by adding molasses to refined white sugar.

Some people recommend the use of honey as an alternative to refined white sugar. However, courtesy of the bees that make it, honey contains enzymes and natural antibiotics that may interfere with the kombucha's microbiology. Most kombucha experts agree that honey can create problems with fermentation, so I don't recommend experimenting. If you want to use honey, don't add it to the boiling water as you would sugar. Instead, wait and add the honey after the tea has cooled down. Ultimately, however, I still strongly recommend using only refined white sugar, especially for beginners.

If you're thinking about using a sugar substitute to avoid refined white sugar, think again. No artificial sweetener will serve as food for the kombucha. The culture, for example, would starve on saccharin, which is made from toluene, a substance that has no food value.

If you're still tempted to avoid sugar, you may be intrigued by the methods of a physician named Meixner. According to author Harald Tietze, Meixner substitutes manna that he makes himself for sugar. Because manna isn't nearly as sweet as sugar, Meixner recommends using three times more manna than sugar. If you're up to it and into traveling, I can tell you where to find manna. It's a dried sweet secretion obtained by cutting into the bark of European ash shrubs and trees, especially varieties of flowering ash (*Fraxinus ornus* and *Fraxinus rotundifolia*) that can be found in southern Europe.

Purified Water

The amount of water that you include in each batch of kombucha tea may be dictated by the size of the glass bowl you use for fermenting. As discussed earlier in this chapter, the general guidelines are to use 2 tea bags and ½ cup of white sugar per quart (liter) of water. It's easy to find glass bowls that will accommodate 2 to 4 quarts of kombucha tea.

Be sure to use only purified water that's free of silt, chlorine, metal residue from water pipes, and chemicals, such as fluorine. While some kombucha enthusiasts have experimented with using distilled water in the past, recent research shows that distilled water produces an inferior kombucha tea because essential minerals are absent.

Gather the Equipment

Now that you have your kombucha culture, tea, white sugar, and purified water, it's time to check your cupboards once more to find the necessary equipment to make kombucha tea. Here is a list of the items you'll need.

A stainless steel pot. You'll need a pot in which to boil the water for the tea; if you prefer, you can also dissolve the sugar and steep the tea in the pot. Choose a pot made of high-quality stainless steel. Nickel is a metal found in stainless steel, and especially when inferior pots are used, remnants of nickel can end up in whatever is being heated. The pot should hold at least 4 quarts (liters) of water. If you want to make more than one batch of tea at a time, I recommend using a commercial-sized pot, which can be found at any restaurant supply store. Remember, it's okay to use a metal pot because the pot will never contain the kombucha culture.

A large glass bowl. You'll need a large bowl in which to store the tea and culture during fermentation. Select a glass bowl (one that holds up to 5 quarts is ideal) without any metal or plastic components, not even on the rim. Plastic, ceramic, or crystal bowls shouldn't be used because the kombucha culture will leach impurities from these products during fermentation. I recommend using a glass Pyrex mixing bowl or a bowl made of tempered glass. The bowl must have a large opening to allow the kombucha culture to unfold and receive an adequate supply of oxygen.

A wooden, ceramic, or glass spoon. Use the spoon to stir the sweetened tea and remove the tea bags after steeping.

A white cotton towel. Use a white cotton kitchen towel to cover the glass bowl that contains the fermenting kombucha tea. The towel will protect the tea from insects and dust. Any clean white or light-colored cotton towel or cloth will do, as will several layers of cheesecloth.

A cotton tea strainer. Use a cotton tea strainer when pouring the fermented tea into glass storage containers. If you don't have a cotton tea strainer, strain the tea by pouring it through cheesecloth or a clean cotton towel.

A funnel. You may need a funnel to pour the fermented tea into glass storage containers. Although I've warned against using plastic near the kombucha culture, it's okay to use a plastic funnel for this step because the tea will pass through the funnel very quickly. There's little chance that the tea will leach any toxins from the plastic during such brief contact. However, *do not use* a metal funnel for this step.

Glass storage containers. Use clear, sterile glass jars or bottles to store the fermented kombucha tea. The number of containers you'll need will depend on the size of the batch and the size of the containers. Top the jars or bottles with corks or plastic lids. Corked clear glass bottles or clean wine bottles work perfectly. Just make sure the containers aren't sealed tightly; the corks or lids must yield to the pressure of the fermenting tea. Even when stored in the refrigerator, the tea will continue to ferment and must have some room to breathe and expand.

Kombucha Tea Ingredients at a Glance

In this chapter, I have kept ingredient guidelines general so you can determine the quantity of tea you wish to brew. In addition to the kombucha culture, here are the proportions I recommend for the tea, water, and white sugar:

- 2 tea bags or 2 teaspoons of loose black, green, or white tea per quart (liter) of purified water
- ½ cup of white sugar per quart (liter) of purified water

The amount of tea you use can be varied according to your own preference. For example, when I brew 3 quarts of tea, I typically use 5 tea bags, not 6 as I recommend in the guidelines. However, don't use less sugar than recommended or you risk starving the kombucha culture during fermentation.

Make the Tea

Brewing kombucha tea isn't an exact science. Variations in taste and appearance will occur because of the uniqueness of each kombucha culture and the subtle differences in each person's preparation methods. Try to follow these instructions as closely as possible, but remember to have fun.

Prepare the "baby." If you're using a newly obtained kombucha baby, remove it from the plastic bag. Gently lay the kombucha in a shallow glass dish and pour any tea that came in the plastic bag into the dish as well. Cover the dish with a clean white cotton towel or cloth, but don't allow the towel to touch the culture. Note that although the kombucha culture needs to be treated with care, it's quite robust and can tolerate this kind of routine handling.

Boil the water. Pour 2 to 4 quarts of purified water into a high-quality stainless steel pot. Put the pot over high heat and bring the water to a boil. Remove the pot from the heat. Note: I decided to begin with only 2 quarts of water the first time I made kombucha tea. I highly recommend this to beginners because this amount is easy to handle and will give you increased confidence. In addition, two-quart glass bowls and storage containers are easy to find.

Add the sugar. While the hot water is in the pot, stir in the white sugar. Use ½ cup of sugar per quart (liter) of water. Stir until the sugar is completely dissolved. Alternatively, return the pot to the heat and boil the water for 2 to 3 minutes until the sugar is completely dissolved.

Add the tea. Now you have a decision to make. You can brew the tea either in the pot or in the glass bowl that you'll use to ferment the kombucha tea. Use 2 teaspoons of loose tea or 2 tea bags for every quart (liter) of water. The amount can be varied to taste or to make the tea weaker or stronger. The recommended steeping time for tea bags is 10 to 15 minutes. The steeping time for loose tea is shorter—3 to 5 minutes. (If you use loose tea, you'll need to strain it, which adds an extra step to the process. If you're a beginner, I advise you to stick with the tried and tested tea bags.)

Remove the tea bags or strain the tea. When the tea is finished brewing, remove the tea bags. If you used loose tea, pour the tea through a sieve, strainer, cheesecloth, or cotton cloth to completely clear the tea of residue. If you like, you can pour the strained tea directly into the glass bowl that you'll use to ferment the kombucha tea, as long as the glass bowl is heatproof.

Let the tea cool. Cover the pot or glass bowl and let the tea cool to lukewarm. It's critical that the tea be cooled completely, as otherwise it could damage or even kill the kombucha culture. Depending on ambient temperature, season, and climate, the cooling-down period could take from a few minutes to a couple of hours.

Pour the tea into the glass bowl. If you brewed the tea in the pot, now is the time to pour the lukewarm tea into the glass bowl that you'll use to ferment the kombucha tea. To avoid breakage, make sure the tea is cool before pouring it into the waiting glass bowl, unless you're using a Pyrex bowl or heatproof bowl. It pays to be patient.

Add some "old" kombucha tea. When the fresh batch of tea is lukewarm and waiting in the glass bowl, take about ½ cup of the previous batch of tea (or the liquid that your first kombucha came in) and pour it into the cooled-down tea.

Place the kombucha on the tea. Gently place the kombucha culture on top of the tea, letting it float on the surface. The darker, rougher side of the kombucha should face down, and the lighter, smoother side should face up. It's okay if some of the tea laps over the top of the kombucha.

Select a safe place for fermentation. Put the bowl of tea in a clean, well-ventilated area. When selecting a location, be sure to avoid direct sunlight and wet, mildewy, or moldy areas near damp walls or potted plants, where spores might get into the fermenting kombucha. For additional tips, see "Choosing the Best Spot for Fermentation," page 61.

Cover the kombucha tea during fermentation. Once you have carried the glass bowl of tea to a safe place for fermentation, cover it with a clean white cotton towel or cloth, using a rubber band or string to secure the towel around the rim of the bowl. Make sure the kombucha tea can get air but that it's protected against insects that might fly or crawl underneath the towel, which shouldn't be allowed to touch the kombucha culture.

Wait while your kombucha tea is ripening. The usual fermenting time is between 7 and 10 days, depending on the desired flavor and sugar content, although some people allow the tea to ferment for up to 14 days. A shorter fermenting period results in a sweeter tea with higher sugar content, and a longer period results in a vinegary tea with little or no sugar. For more information, see "Deciding How Long to Ferment the Tea," page 61.

Harvest the tea when it's ready. After the tea has fermented for 7 to 14 days, put the bowl of fermenting tea on the kitchen counter. Wash your hands well. Remove the cotton towel. Remove the culture and gently separate the parent kombucha from the baby. You now have two cultures and can double your efforts. For tips on how to store the kombucha cultures until you brew your next batch or find a new home for the baby, see "Storing the Kombucha Culture" on page 60.

Store the tea. Pour the fresh kombucha tea through the cotton tea strainer (or strain the tea through a clean white cloth) into clean glass bottles that can be corked or loosely sealed. You may need to use a funnel for this step; if so, it's okay to use a plastic funnel because the tea will be in contact with the plastic for only a short time. Don't seal the glass bottles tightly because the tea will continue to ferment, potentially creating enough pressure to cause a problem. You don't want to burst your bubbly!

Stored in glass containers in the refrigerator, kombucha tea will keep for a few weeks. Then, you'll be ready to brew your next batch. Note: Always save one cup of the most recent batch to use when brewing your next batch. You may want to store this small amount of tea right in your fermentation bowl. For more information, see "Caring for the Fermentation Bowl," below.

Create Your Own Favorite Blends at Home

Home-brewed kombucha tea lends itself to blending with other beverages, such as green tea or raspberry tea. Or try combining equal parts of kombucha tea with apple juice; the result is a blend that children particularly enjoy. Another option is to stir in flavored syrups, such as berry syrups. Want to be really adventurous? Throw a kombucha tea party and have guests create their own blended beverages.

More Keys to Kombucha Success

While making kombucha tea isn't difficult, it's obviously quite different than making other types of tea. After all, kombucha tea uniquely requires the use of a live culture. While I have already touched briefly on some of the following points, I think they deserve emphasis. Here is additional background that may contribute to your brewing success.

Caring for the Fermentation Bowl

Some kombucha experts prefer to rinse the fermentation bowl completely after making each batch; they then add a portion of the old tea to each new batch. Here, I want to offer an alternative. As far as I can determine, both methods bring equally good results.

I prefer to leave a small amount (about one cup) of tea right in the fermentation bowl, where a bit of yeast sediment naturally forms while each batch is brewing. Leave the tea and sediment in the fermentation bowl and store it there until you make your next batch. After you've used this method to make three or four batches, clean out the fermentation bowl by rinsing it with hot water. At that time, throw out the yeast sediment. If you store a little bit of the tea and the sediment in the fermentation bowl like this, you won't need to include additional tea from the previous batch.

Storing the Kombucha Culture

Some kombucha experts recommend rinsing the kombucha culture under cold water before storing it; however, a kombucha doesn't have to be rinsed before being reused. After I have finished brewing a batch of kombucha tea and am ready to store the kombucha, I don't wash it. I simply separate the new culture from the original, pour the fresh tea into clean containers, and put one cup of the old tea and the kombucha culture in my glass fermentation bowl. Stored in the refrigerator, the kombucha culture will keep for up to three months.

A healthy kombucha baby can be sealed in a glass container with some kombucha tea and stored in the refrigerator for three to six months. Over this period, the kombucha will turn the tea into vinegar. When you use this vinegary kombucha for a new batch of tea, you won't need to ferment it as long as usual because a kombucha baby will grow very quickly. It's customary to store a kombucha baby in a plastic bag for short-term transport, but since exposure to plastic isn't ideal, the baby would benefit from being stored in a glass container before and after transport.

People who are serious about having a kombucha backup might be interested in learning about additional, although less common, storage methods. Though some experts caution against freezing a kombucha culture because of possible crystallization damage, there are reports of people who have successfully stored kombucha cultures in their freezer for up to five years. If you wish, you could give this a try.

It also appears that the kombucha culture can successfully be dehydrated, which may be ideal for shipping purposes. I haven't tried it, but Harald Tietze reports that a kombucha culture can be dried at 92 degrees F (33 degrees C). Note, however, that the culture shouldn't be exposed to direct sunlight, nor should it be put in a microwave oven for drying or any other purpose; this would kill the kombucha. If you want to dry a kombucha culture, I advise that you purchase a professional dehydrator for this purpose.

To revive the dried kombucha, use it to make a batch of tea with the following ingredients: ½ quart (liter) of purified water, ⅓ cup (80 grams) of white sugar, 2 tea bags, and 1 teaspoon of boiled cider vinegar. Ferment the first batch of tea using the dried kombucha for at least 15 days.

Choosing the Best Spot for Fermentation

Identifying a safe area in your home in which to ferment kombucha tea is as important as any of the other steps in making the tea. The fermenting kombucha needs an optimal growing environment. Choose a spot in your attic or basement or any other suitable room that's neither too cold nor too warm. I successfully ferment my kombucha tea in the basement, but any place in your house or apartment will do, provided it's not in direct sunlight, has sufficient airflow, and isn't hot during the day. That means that most kitchen shelves or bedrooms would work just fine.

Kombucha tea is best left undisturbed during fermentation. I always affix a yellow sticker that says "Do not touch" to my fermentation bowl so that unsuspecting family members will be warned against moving it.

Deciding How Long to Ferment the Tea

If the weather conditions are favorable, you'll probably find that 8 days of fermentation is ideal. If the storage area is hot, 7 days may be sufficient. If the storage area is cold or you prefer a tea with a more acidic taste—or less residual sugar—allow the tea to ferment for 10 days. If the tea is left to ferment for 10 to 14 days, the sugar content should be almost entirely consumed by the bacteria and yeast in the kombucha culture.

The longer the tea ferments, the more vinegary it will taste. If your first batch of tea is too strong, dilute it by adding purified water or fresh tea. For your next batch, shorten the fermentation period or experiment with the sugar content.

You may accidentally discover kombucha vinegar if you allow the tea to ferment for 15 days or store it in the refrigerator for a long time. Don't worry. The kombucha tea becomes a viable vinegar that you can use just like any other vinegar. Feel free to add it to salads and other dishes.

Planning Your Kombucha Tea Program

At this point you may be wondering how many batches of kombucha tea you'll need to ferment simultaneously to maintain a program. For beginners, a good program consists of drinking two shot glasses full of kombucha tea on an empty stomach every morning. My own program involves drinking ½ cup of tea in the morning and ½ cup again before retiring. So that both my wife and I can maintain this program, we usually have two batches fermenting at a time. This allows us to have some left over to share with family, friends, neighbors, and pets. I think you'll quickly be able to determine how much kombucha tea to make depending on your family's needs.

The Longevity of a Kombucha

Your kombucha culture came to you from uncountable generations of predecessors. If it's treated correctly, the kombucha won't die. Yet, I notice that the longer a kombucha culture lives and produces babies, the more old and weary it appears to grow. Once you're familiar with the kombucha, you'll be able to recognize the telltale signs of age. A kombucha culture also may age if it's kept inactive for too long either in the refrigerator or in an area with little air. It will start to look frayed, spotty, and dark.

The good news, however, is that simply by using your kombucha culture to make kombucha tea, you'll be providing yourself with a never-ending supply of kombucha babies. So perhaps it's not necessary to investigate the kombucha's lifespan too closely. If all has gone well, you'll have many new kombucha babies and can safely throw your aging kombucha away. It has served its purpose and outlived its usefulness.

From all the expert evidence I've gathered to date, it appears conclusive that every kombucha baby has the same potency as its parent. So, without further ado, go ahead and use the baby when making your next batch of tea.

When a Kombucha Becomes Moldy

Sometimes mold will form on top of a kombucha culture during fermentation. This happened to me once when I used two different kombucha cultures in the same batch of tea. I had harvested this very large batch with two other batches. While the other two were fine, the mixed batch had grayish-green mold spots on the fully developed kombucha baby. During the fermenting process, the bowl with the double batch wasn't sealed as tightly as the other two batches, which may have contributed to the mold growth.

Some authors say it's safe to wash the mold off and continue as usual. They suggest rinsing the mother kombucha thoroughly under cold water

Kombucha Tea That Bubbles Like Champagne

When the tea has fermented and you remove the kombucha culture from the tea's surface, the liquid will look much the same as it did when you first stored it away. However, you'll notice that something exciting happens when you start to pour the tea from the fermentation bowl into glass bottles for storage. The first time I poured my kombucha tea, I was stunned. The tea foamed and bubbled like newly opened champagne.

That first day, I poured myself a large glass of my newly harvested kombucha tea and drank it with gusto. I was drinking a tea that tasted like French champagne, the best drink in the world. By the time my wife came home to taste the tea, the bubbles had settled, and we were drinking tea that tasted like apple cider. Ah, but that first drink on harvest day is a treat to look forward to. In fact, if you have a large family, you may end up drinking all the champagne-like kombucha tea at this time.

To make kombucha champagne, follow the recipe on page 56, using orange pekoe tea and ½ cup of refined white sugar per quart (liter) of purified water. Cover the tea with a clean white cotton towel and allow it to ferment in a dark place, preferably high up on a shelf in the basement near the air vent, for 8 days. Pour the fermented tea into a champagne glass, straining it through a cotton tea strainer. Watch the bubbles rise and drink immediately. Every time I make kombucha tea this way, it tastes just like champagne.

to remove all signs of mold, then rinsing it in cider vinegar. This cleansing treatment should fully restore the health of the kombucha and make it ready for the next batch of tea.

However, I prefer to be cautious and advise others to be the same. My motto is "When in doubt, throw it out." When I saw mold on the kombucha culture, I trashed the entire batch of tea as well as the kombucha. While most molds are harmless, some may be dangerous, and I wasn't taking any chances. Follow my lead: if you see mold on the kombucha, throw away the culture and the tea and start fresh with a new kombucha.

When a Kombucha Dies

If a kombucha dies, chances are it has been exposed to nicotine from some form of tobacco. According to Harald Tietze, this is the case in 50 percent of kombucha deaths. Other common causes of death include the use of honey, which has antibiotic constituents that can slowly kill off a kombucha, or starvation. A kombucha culture will starve to death if it's deprived of sugar. For this reason, never use less sugar than I recommend in the general guidelines. See sidebar, page 56.

If your kombucha culture has died and you don't have another one to keep you going, return to the source where you got your first kombucha. If that's not possible, see Resources (page 79) for further guidance. While you're in between kombucha cultures, you may want to use commercial kombucha drinks, extracts, medicinal tonics, or tinctures. See Professional Brews, page 68.

FAQ

Q: **Where can I get a kombucha culture?**

A: Check Resources (page 79) for suppliers or see your local natural food store or natural health publication for a reliable source. Only buy or accept a kombucha culture from someone you trust. It's important to have a healthy and viable kombucha for breeding babies and making the tea.

Q: **Can I ferment kombucha tea without using refined white sugar?**

A: My advice is to stick to the instructions provided in this chapter. I particularly recommend that beginners use white sugar. Some people try molasses, dark sugars, or honey when making kombucha tea. Experiment at your own risk, and only if you're an advanced user. And remember: the sugar in the tea isn't there for you. It's there to feed the bacteria and yeast, which would die without it. If you don't want to consume sugar, simply let the tea ferment for 14 days. After that time, there will be no (or very little) sugar remaining when you drink the tea.

Q: **Can I store or ferment the kombucha tea in plastic or metal?**

A: According to reliable research, a kombucha leaches potentially harmful compounds from plastics and metals and incorporates them into its structure, passing the toxins on to its babies and the tea. For this reason, avoid plastic and metal utensils and containers. In addition, don't use lead crystal bowls (the lead is toxic). I recommend using Pyrex glass.

Q: **What type of container should I use for fermenting the tea?**

A: For the best results, ferment kombucha tea in a glass bowl. When you use a bowl, you'll get a moderate-sized kombucha; however, if you use a glass lasagne pan or casserole, you'll get a much larger culture. Also, when it's placed in a bowl, the culture has more exposure to the tea mixture and to oxygen. Jars and cylinders shouldn't be used because they're too narrow.

Q: Can I cut a kombucha in half and make two batches of tea at once?

A: Yes, you can even cut it in thirds and make three batches. As long as you follow the instructions in this chapter, the tea should turn out fine. Incidentally, I have started one batch by using only a small portion of a kombucha culture. It worked well. The fragmented kombucha parent gave birth to a healthy, full-grown baby.

Q: Can kombucha tea make a kombucha baby all on its own?

A: Yes. A kombucha baby can start to form on top of kombucha tea if the tea is left in a warm spot for an extended period of time. To prevent kombucha tea from making a new culture, store it in the refrigerator.

Q: How will I know if my tea turned out right?

A: If you follow my instructions, nothing should go wrong. After a successful brew, a kombucha baby should be formed. It can be on top of the mother or on top of the tea if the mother sank to the bottom of the bowl. See the next question.

Q: My kombucha sank to the bottom of the bowl. Is it dead?

A: If there's less oxygen in the kombucha mother, it may sink to the bottom. As long as it produced a healthy baby, all should be well.

Q: My kombucha baby is very thin. Is this normal?

A: Yes. Kombucha cultures come in all shapes and sizes. Under cool conditions, a kombucha mother may produce a thin baby, but the baby should still be viable. To encourage more growth, put the fermentation bowl in a warm environment: 72 to 86 degrees F (22 to 30 degrees C) is optimal. Alternatively, try adding more sugar to increase growth during the winter months.

Q: My kombucha culture is covered in mold. What should I do?

A: The safest thing to do is throw it out and start fresh. Perhaps the kombucha you received was contaminated. Or fruit flies and other contaminants may have gotten into the fermenting tea. To avoid mold in the future, make sure the fermentation bowl is properly covered, which means the mixture should be protected but getting sufficient oxygen. Keep the bowl away from plants, fruits, vegetables, compost, and garbage. I repeat, "When in doubt, throw it out!"

Q: If a kombucha dries out, can I still use it?

A: If the kombucha wasn't in contact with contaminants, such as food particles, fruit flies, metals, or plastics, you should be able to revive it. Simply rinse the culture with kombucha tea or cider vinegar. Let it soak for fifteen minutes in the tea or vinegar. Then, proceed with a new batch of tea according to my instructions, adding a bit of the tea or vinegar you used for rinsing the kombucha culture. If your new tea doesn't turn out, the kombucha may be dead. Throw it out and get another.

Q: Is there a right way to throw away a kombucha culture?

A: The right way is to simply throw the old kombucha in the garbage. I'm more concerned about the wrong way to dispose of a kombucha, which can be disastrous to your plumbing. Never discard a kombucha culture by flushing it down the toilet or putting it down the sink drain. It may attach somewhere and grow, eventually clogging up the drainpipes.

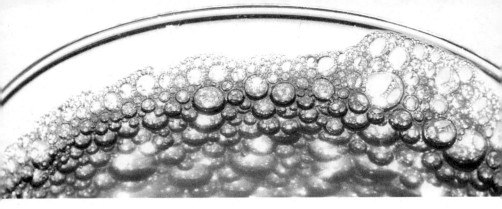

Chapter Six
The Professional Brews

Tea ceremonies, you say, aren't your style and the kitchen isn't your favorite place? Relax. Even if you aren't interested in brewing your own kombucha tea, you can still benefit from drinking commercially brewed kombucha tea or using other products, such as extracts, tinctures, and tonics, that are also available. A growing number of companies are now producing and marketing kombucha products. You can find these teas and other products in pharmacies and natural food stores; they also can also be purchased on the Internet.

I made several interesting discoveries when I did some research on the current selections of commercial kombucha teas. These brews often feature unusual and exotic flavor combinations. In addition, they may contain less sugar than home-brewed teas. If sugar content is a concern for you, check the nutrition facts on the label for the amount of sugar per serving.

Following is a list of some of the teas I explored (I was even able to sample some of them), along with some background I found about each manufacturer. You may recognize some of these brand names next time you peruse refrigerated bottled drinks at your favorite natural food store. For each company's contact information, see Resources (page 79).

Enlightened Organic Raw Kombucha. Made by Millennium Products of California, this kombucha drink is available at many natural food stores in the United States and Canada. Varieties include original, citrus, gingerade, and multi-green. The company's principal, G. T. Dave, started bottling kombucha in 1995, which also happens to be the year the first edition of this book came out. The company includes a promise on the product label, stating it will remain committed to "expanding gradually and organically, never sacrificing quality for the sake of profits." I tasted this brew and liked it. It looks, fizzes, and tastes like home-brewed kombucha tea.

Éternité Kombucha. This is a commercial kombucha drink that "sparkles." From a company called Crudessence in Montreal, Quebec, this product is available in several flavors.

High Country Kombucha. Sold throughout the United States, this probiotic fermented tea is brewed in the Colorado Rocky Mountains using only pure spring water. Bottled in amber glass to protect it from ultraviolet light, the tea is available in a number of varieties, including aloe, chai, and wild root (similar to root beer).

Katalyst Kombucha. Based in Greenfield, Massachusetts, this company bottles several raw and organic kombucha drinks that are sold on the East Coast. Some unique flavorings include Cordyceps mushrooms, blue-green algae, and schizandra berry (the berry is used in traditional Chinese medicine).

Kombucha Brooklyn. Founded by "kombuchman" Eric Childs in Brooklyn, New York, the company bases its formula on a combination of black, green, and white teas. The bottled drink is available in multiple flavors; the tea is also sold on tap in more than a dozen Brookyln and New York City eateries and markets.

Kombucha Wonder Drink. This effervescent drink is available in bottles and cans and comes in a wide range of flavors. American-made in Oregon, this drink has a refreshing kombucha tea taste.

Pronatura Original Kombucha Drink. The first commercial kombucha product distributor in North America was Pronatura. The company sells a commercial kombucha tea that's prepared in Germany according to Rudolf Sklenar's original kombucha tea formula. A physician, Sklenar used his formula to treat cancer patients (see page 36). Pronatura has sold the product for more than forty years, during which time there have been no safety problems. The company's staff assures customers that the tea is not only safe but also tastes great. Kombucha expert Betsy Pryor echoes this comment. She describes the tea as delicious and confirms that Pronatura's kombucha tea is "alive," meaning that traditional methods are used to assure the best fermentation.

ThéBÜ Kombucha Tea. This organic kombucha tea is manufactured by Makana Beverages, a company founded by three surfing entrepreneurs in Hawaii who have expanded their kombucha tea business into California. *Makana* is a Hawaiian word that means "gift," and the drink is the company's gift to kombucha lovers. Flavors include lavender, melon, tangerine, and tropical.

Tonica Kombucha. This Toronto-based company offers kombucha drinks made with filtered water, the kombucha culture, fermented organic cane sugar, and fermented organic green and white tea. Flavors include blueberry, ginger, mango, and peach. I tried the mango variety and found it refreshingly tasty and very lively.

Yogi Green Tea Kombucha Teabags. I have no knowledge of the efficacy of this product as compared with the live kombucha drink, but I can say that the tea is flavorful. I do, however, prefer and recommend active kombucha tea over any kind of tea that includes dried kombucha.

Beyond Tea

Tea is one of the most common retail kombucha products available. Other kombucha-based products, however, are also marketed. One example is pressed extract, a biological medicine made from the symbiosis itself. Pronatura describes its extract as a concentrated liquid that promotes general health, well-being, and detoxification, just like the tea. Another product is kombucha tincture. Helmut Golz reports that kombucha tinctures can have a positive effect on infections with or without fever, diverse metabolic disorders, allergic reactions, sleeplessness, fatigue, and general debility. The tinctures apparently keep for three months and can easily be self-administered.

One Internet source for kombucha products is the Happy Herbalist website (see Resources, page 79). The site advertises such products as kombucha extracts and a homeopathic kombucha liquid formula. The Happy Herbalist also is a source for a kombucha starter kit and offers kombucha lore, cautions, and tips for home brewers.

Kefiplant and Chantale Houle

Now it's time to share an encouraging tale of an entrepreneur who is interested in improving people's health. Chantale Houle, a bright and industrious French

Canadian, loves kombucha tea and has revolutionized the way kombucha is used medicinally. Following the sale of her family's oak flooring business, Houle had the resources to pursue her dreams by forming Kefiplant, a company that produces and distributes kombucha formulations to the food, beverage, supplement, cosmetic, and agricultural industries. She told me her story over dinner in Anaheim, California.

Houle earned a bachelor's degree from Quebec's Laval University in 1993. She studied phytotherapy and microbiology, eventually concentrating on the fermentation of symbioses of bacteria and yeasts. Houle focused her research on the restorative nature of kombucha tea, and she developed worldwide contacts with experts who worked in the field of fermentation. One of her contacts, a French scientist named Sergi Rollan, became a valued source and, eventually, her partner at Kefiplant.

Houle incorporated Kefiplant near Montreal in her hometown of Drummondville, Quebec, in 2004 and has since won many accolades and awards. She told me that as a result of her research, she initially offered purified kombucha for free to nearby farmers for treating sick animals. The farmers were reportedly astounded by the recovery rates of animals they had given up for lost. Word of the lady from Drummondville and her kombucha quickly spread.

Over the years, Kefiplant has grown as a manufacturer of kombucha and other health products. The company built a large laboratory in which to purify their kombucha formulas and make them available for commercial distribution throughout the North American health food industry. Kefiplant's mission is to be a world leader in the production of organic bioavailable phytocompounds and nutrients from fermented botanicals.

Sergi Rollan's Kefir Grain

Sergi Rollan is Houle's scientist partner and director of research at Kefiplant. He attended the French National Center for Scientific Research, where he earned several degrees during the late 1970s and 1980s. He obtained a doctor of medicine degree, a nutritional and dietary research degree, a research degree in acupuncture, a research degree in phytotherapy and homeopathy, and a pharmaceutical doctorate. In addition to his work with Kefiplant, Rollan is a scientific and medical consultant for a number of well-known French laboratories and companies.

Having researched and traveled in search of the purified kombucha for over twenty years, Rollan finally tracked down what he calls the "original" kefir grain, a microorganism of yeast and bacteria symbiosis. Why call it a kefir grain and not kombucha grain? Using Rollan's own words: "Add milk and get kefir; add water and get kombucha." (Kefir is a beverage made of fermented cow's milk; you can read about it in my book *Kefir Rediscovered!)*

Rollan and the experts at Kefiplant claim that most commercial and domestic kombuchas have weakened or mutated over time, losing some significant yeasts and bacteria while developing other wild strains of yeasts and bacteria that weren't present in the original symbiosis. That's why Rollan says that kombucha tea made at home doesn't have the properties of kombucha tea made hundreds of years ago. I can't confirm his claims at this time, but I was told that Rollan is planning clinical trials and will publish his findings in a peer-reviewed journal. I can hardly wait.

A Strain of Kombucha Like the Ancients Used

According to Rollan and Kefiplant, their research involves the science of phylogeny (also called phylogenesis), which is the evolution and history of a genetically related group of organisms. Research has confirmed the genetic integrity of Kefiplant's kefir grain, which the company claims is more potent than the common kombucha culture used by most commercial and home brewers today.

Kefiplant uses a proprietary fermentation process. Instead of using a "mother" culture whose "babies" are passed on for reproduction, the company's process utilizes the original culture for every batch of kombucha medicinals, thus ensuring the purest fermentation. Kefiplant claims that its "kefir kombucha" is an organic, vegan, raw, nutrient-packed kombucha like the Asian kombucha of ancient times.

Because minerals and antioxidants are generally difficult for the body to digest and absorb, Kefiplant's patented fermentation process renders minerals and antioxidants into a predigested form that the body can easily assimilate. For example, Kefiplant claims that when black tea is fermented to make kombucha, iron is the most significant mineral converted to a bioavailable form. Analysis shows that because of Kefiplant's unique fermentation process, its kombucha has more bioavailable antioxidants than other brands.

Kefiplant Trademarks

Kefiplant has created several trademarked fermented botanicals based on the original kombucha formula made from its kefir grain. Following is a list of Kefiplant's trademarked processes and products:

KefiTech. KefiTech is Kefiplant's overall trademark for the patented fermentation process based on the kefir grain. The fermented formulas produce a variety of healthful botanicals that are beneficial to humans and animals alike.

KefiActive. A supplemental form of a fermented botanical that contains water-soluble bioactive compounds, each KefiActive formula contains bioavailable micronutrients and nanonutrients, such as organic acids, beneficial yeasts and bacteria, enzymes, vitamins, and minerals that are all released by fermentation. Kefiplant claims that its formulas are antimicrobial and don't require preservatives, which I find is true of most other commercial kombucha products and even homemade kombucha tea.

KefiApéro. Used in aperitifs and digestives that are taken before or after meals to promote digestion, KefiApéro comes in such flavors as anise, ginger, holy basil, and peppermint. All varieties are mildly sweet and acidic and contain 2 to 4 percent alcohol. They can be mixed with vodka or gin.

KefiFood. Used in place of harmful chemicals to enhance foods, KefiFood can be used to reduce salt content and extend the shelf life of prepared foods. It also adds antioxidants and nutrients (such as polyphenols, organic acids, B vitamins, amino acids, minerals, and so forth) to food formulations.

KefiNutra. Used in supplements, KefiNutra contains bioavailable phytocompounds and beneficial micronutrients and nanonutrients. It's designed to rejuvenate and restore health, increase vital energy, improve digestion, and support a healthy intestinal tract.

KefiSkin. Used in topical body care, KefiSkin provides powerful antimicrobial ingredients for alleviating skin problems, such as acne, eczema, fungal infections, and psoriasis. It's well known that kombucha tea and kefir are good for the skin. Kefiplant claims that the nutrients in the KefiSkin formula also help to heal burns.

KefiViva. Used to enhance beverages, KefiViva is designed to support healthy digestion, cultivate good intestinal flora, and provide bioavailable antioxidants. KefiViva can be added to bottled (carbonated or noncarbonated, raw or pasteurized) juices or herbal drinks to create fermentation.

A Variety of Kombucha Tonics

Kefiplant's medicinal products are distributed in Canada solely by TallGrass of Vancouver, British Columbia. As I learned from Matthew Breech, TallGrass president and CEO, Kefiplant provides the basis for a variety of therapeutic liquid energizers. The revitalizing tonics contain bioavailable phytocompounds and enzymes, vitamins, friendly yeast and bacteria, and other micronutrients that contribute to a medicinal synergy, all with the added benefit of including zero calories.

Kefiplant's trademarked tonics are sold through natural food stores in Canada. All of the tonics are based on Kefiplant's kefir grain research, and the company claims the tonics are as live and active as any homemade kombucha tea, and possibly more so. That's why I feel a mention of these products belongs in this book, although I won't offer in-depth details about their medicinal values. Following is a list of available tonics:

Botanica KefiActive Kombucha Revitalizing Tonic. Made of kombucha-fermented black tea, this tonic contains active cultures and is designed to revitalize the body, improve digestion, detoxify, and maintain a healthy intestinal tract.

Botanica KefiActive Fermented Astragalus Immune Tonic. Made from fermented astragalus tea, this tonic is designed to help combat frequent colds.

Botanica KefiActive Fermented Echinacea Formula. Made from fermented echinacea tea, this tonic is designed to fight off infection, particularly upper respiratory tract infections.

Botanica KefiActive Fermented Holy Basil Formula. Featuring bioavailable ocimumoside and other significant phytocompounds found in holy basil, this tonic is designed to alleviate mood swings and mild depression.

Botanica KefiActive Oregano Antimocrobial. Made with oregano tea fermented from *Origanum vulgare* leaves, this tonic is designed to help maintain a healthy intestinal tract. The literature claims that fermentation transforms significant phytocompounds in oregano, offering effective oregano in whole-food form.

Botanica KefiActive Passionflower Sleep Aid. Made with fermented passionflower tea, this tonic is sold as a sleep aid to relieve restlessness and insomnia.

Glossary

Acidosis. Acidosis describes a state of excessive acidity in body fluids.

Alkalinity. Alkalinity refers to a solution's ability to neutralize acids. An alkaline solution has a pH greater than seven.

Alkalosis. Alkalosis describes a state of excessive alkalinity in body fluids.

Antioxidant. Found in plant foods and certain vitamins, antioxidants inhibit oxidation and fight free radicals, supporting health and longevity.

Aperitif. An aperitif is an alcoholic drink used as an appetizer before a meal.

Astragalus membranaceus. Also known as *Astragalus propinquus*, *Astragalus membranaceus* is an herbal medicinal used in traditional Chinese medicine. It reportedly has antiaging and antiviral properties, and there are some indications that it may have potential benefits for the immune system, the heart, and the liver. It may also be valuable as an adjunct to cancer therapy. *Astragalus membranaceus* is one of many species of astragalus.

Bifidobacteria. Bifidobacteria are a type of bacteria that live in the intestines of mammals. Some strands of bifidobacteria are used as probiotics (see page 25).

Catechins. Found in tea, particularly in green tea, catechins are health-supporting antioxidants. In black tea, catechins become theaflavins (polyphenols, see page 78), which also offer positive health effects. Orange-colored teas contain greater amounts of theaflavins.

Colibacillosis. A disease caused by *Escherichia coli* in humans and other species, colibacillosis symptoms include diarrhea.

Digestive. A digestive is a substance that aids digestion.

Diuretic. A diuretic is any substance that promotes the formation of urine by the kidneys and increases the amount of urination to expel liquid from the body.

Edema. Edema is a condition in which abnormally large volumes of fluid accumulate in the body's circulatory system or in tissues between cells.

Glucaric acid. While some kombucha experts believe glucuronic acid (see below) is present in kombucha tea, recent research confirms the presence of glucaric acid, which helps eliminate the glucuronic acid conjugates that are produced by the liver. Therefore, glucaric acid probably makes the liver more efficient. In addition, glucaric acid, which is found in fruits and vegetables, is being explored as a cancer-preventive agent.

Gluconate. Gluconate is an ion of gluconic acid (see below).

Gluconic acid. A naturally occurring organic compound that regulates acidity, gluconic acid is formed from the sugars in honey, kombucha tea, and wine.

Glucuronic acid. A sugar acid formed by the oxidation of glucose to a carboxyl group, glucuronic acid is conjugated in the liver, forming glucuronides, which are excreted in the urine. Glucuronic acid is instrumental in detoxifying the body. Kombucha researchers disagree about whether or not glucuronic acid is present in kombucha tea; earlier research indicated it was present, while more recent research points to the presence of glucaric acid (see above), and not glucuronic acid.

Glycolysis. The breakdown of glucose to pyruvate, glycolysis is a metabolic process that releases usable energy. It takes place in nearly all living cells.

Homeopathy. Homeopathy is a complementary disease-treatment system in which a patient is given minute doses of natural substances that in larger doses would produce symptoms of the disease itself. Homeopathy has a huge following, and there are many homeopathic practitioners. There also are many scientific critics who consider homeopathy no more useful than a placebo, and the effectiveness of homeopathy has been in dispute since its inception.

Kefir. Kefir is a fermented beverage made with cow's milk and a symbiosis of yeast and bacteria.

Kefir grain. A symbiotic culture of yeast and bacteria, kefir grain is used to make kefir. According to Kefiplant, the same symbiosis, when put into tea instead of milk, can be used to make kombucha tea.

Lactic acid. A colorless organic acid produced by muscles and found in sour milk, lactic acid is used in fermentation, as a preservative, and in dyeing.

Lactobacillus. A major group of lactic acid bacteria that convert lactose and other sugars to lactic acid, lactobacillus are used in the manufacture of yogurt, cheeses, sauerkraut, and other fermented foods.

Nanonutrients. In food technology, nanonutrients are nutrients that are greatly reduced in size to facilitate uptake by the cells for medicinal purposes.

Ocimumoside. A component of holy basil, ocimumoside is widely used as a medicinal herbal.

Pathogen. A pathogen is any disease-causing agent, especially a virus, bacterium, or other microorganism.

pH. The measure of acidity or alkalinity in a solution, pH is represented by a numerical scale in which seven is neutral, with lower numbers indicating acidity and higher numbers indicating alkalinity.

Phagocyte. A phagocyte is a white blood cell in the body's bloodstream and tissues that engulfs and ingests foreign particles, cell waste material, and bacteria.

Phylogenesis. See phylogeny.

Phylogeny. Phylogeny is the study of the evolution and history of a genetically related group of organisms, such as a species. It's also called phylogenesis.

Phytocompounds. Phytocompounds are bioactive combinations of medicinal and herbal plants.

Phytofermentation. A term used by Kefiplant, phytofermentation uses plants as active ingredients in the fermenting process.

Phytotherapy. Phytotherapy is the use of plant products for medicinal purposes.

Polyphenols. Polyphenols are plant-based chemicals and antioxidants that scavenge free radicals and thereby tone the body and prevent premature aging. Rich sources include white tea and green tea (see catechins, page 76).

Probiotic. A preparation that includes beneficial bacteria, a probiotic is taken orally to restore the healthful balance of bacteria in the gut.

Protozoan. A protozoan is a tiny organism that's usually single celled and uses organic carbon as a source of energy.

SCOBY. An acronym that refers to the kombucha culture, SCOBY stands for "symbiotic colony of bacteria and yeast."

Symbiosis. A symbiosis is a permanent or long-term association of organisms living together for mutual benefit.

Usnic acid. Found in lichen and also reportedly in the kombucha culture, usnic acid has many medicinal properties. It's an analgesic, anti-inflammatory, antioxidant, and antiviral. It also is known to inhibit the growth of protozoans and disrupt mitosis (cell division).

Resources

Books
Book Publishing Company
bookpubco.com
1-931-964-3571

Kombucha Starter Kits
Cultures for Health
culturesforhealth.com
Toll-free: 1-800-962-1959

Happy Herbalist
happyherbalist.com
1-919-267-6776
Toll-free: 1-888-425-8827
Contact: Ed Kasper

Kombucha Exchange Worldwide
kombu.de/suche2.htm#uk
Contact: Günther Frank

Makers of Professional Brews
Crudessence
Maker of Éternité Kombucha.
crudessence.com
1-514-271-0333
Toll-free: 1-877-271-0940

Golden Temple of Oregon
Maker of Yogi Green Tea Kombucha.
yogiproducts.com
1-800-YOGI-TEA

High Country Kombucha
hckombu.com
1-970-328-1827

Katalyst Kombucha
katalystkombucha.com
1-413-773-9700

Kefiplant
Manufacturer of fermented plant and
kombucha extracts.
kefiplant.com
1-819-477-2345
Contact: Suzanne Stoeckle

Kombucha Brooklyn
kombuchabrooklyn.com
Contact: Eric Childs

Kombucha Wonder Drink
wonderdrink.com
1-877-224-7331

Makana Beverages
Maker of ThéBü Kombucha Tea.
thebukombucha.com
1-805-981-8638
Toll-free: 1-808-936-6000
Contact: Ryan Mason

Millennium Products
Maker of Organic Raw Kombucha.
synergydrinks.com
Toll-free: 1-877-735-8423

Pronatura
Maker and distributor of kombucha tea,
extracts, and capsules.
pronaturainc.com
1-847-718-0899
Toll-free: 1-800-555-7580
Contact: Andre Mehrabian

TallGrass
Distributor of kombucha medicinal tonics.
tallgrass.ca
1-604-709-0101
1-800-616-5900
Contact: Matthew Breech

Tonica Kombucha
tonicakombucha.com
1-416-901-5888

Bibliography

Ahmadjian, Vernon, and Surinda Paracer. *Symbiosis.* Hanover, NH: University Press, 1986.

Chaitow, Leon, and Natasha Trenves. *Probiotics.* Wellingborough, England: Thorsons, 1990.

Fasching, Rosina. *Le Champignon de Longue vie Combucha.* Steyr, Austria: W. Ennsthaler, 1989.

Fasching, Rosina. *Tea Fungus Kombucha.* Steyr, Austria: W. Ennsthaler, 1987.

Fischer, William L. *How to Fight Cancer & Win.* Vancouver, BC: Alive Books, 1987.

Frank, Günther W. *Kombucha: Das Teepilz-Getränk.* Steyr, Austria: W. Ennsthaler, 1991.

Golz, Helmut. *Kombucha: Ein Altes Teeheilmittel.* Munich: Ariston Verlag, 1992.

Haard, Richard, and Karen Haard. *Foraging for Edible Wild Mushrooms.* Seattle: Homestead Book Co., 1980.

Haard, Richard, and Karen Haard. *Poisonous & Hallucinogenic Mushrooms.* Seattle: Homestead Book Co., 1980.

Harnisch, Günther. *Kombucha: Geballte Heilkraft aus der Natur.* Beitigheim-Bissingen, Germany: Turm-Verlag, 1991.

Hobbs, Christopher. *Kombucha Manchurian Tea Mushroom: The Essential Guide.* Santa Cruz, CA: Botanica Press, 1995.

Hobbs, Christopher. *Medicinal Mushrooms.* Santa Cruz, CA: Botanica Press, 1995.

Pryor, Betsy, and Sanford Holst. *Kombucha Phenomenon.* Sherman Oaks, CA: Sierra Sunrise Books, 1995.

Read, Clark P. *Parasitism and Symbiology.* New York: Ronald Press, 1970.

Rossmoore, Harold W. *The Microbes, Our Unseen Friends.* Detroit: Wayne State University Press, 1976.

Stevenson, Greta. *The Biology of Fungi, Bacteria, and Viruses.* New York: American Elsevier Publishing, 1970.

Tietze, Harald W. *Kombucha: The Miracle Fungus.* Bermagui South, NSW, Australia: Gateway Books, 1994.

Index

Page references for sidebars appear in *italics*.

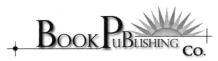

books that educate, inspire, and empower
To find your favorite vegetarian and soyfood products online, visit:
www.healthy-eating.com

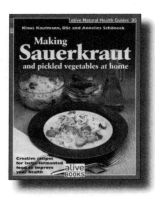

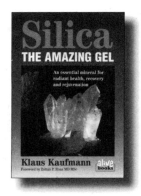

Making Sauerkraut
Klaus Kaufmann, DSc, and
Annelies Schöneck
978-1-55312-037-7 $11.95

Silica
The Amazing Gel
Klaus Kaufmann, DSc
978-0-920470-30-5 $11.95

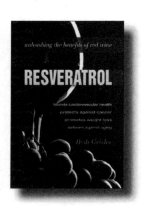

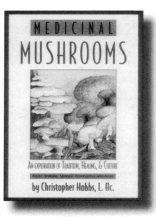

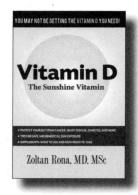

Resveratrol
Beth Geisler
978-157067-242-2 $9.95

Medicinal Mushrooms
Christopher Hobbs, LAc
978-1-57067-143-2 $19.95

Vitamin D
Zoltan Rona, MD, MSc
978-0-920470-82-4 $9.95